POCKET CONSULT

Rheumatology

G. V. Campion
MD, MRCP
Lecturer,
University of Bristol

A. St J. Dixon
MD, FRCP
Consultant Physician,
Royal United Hospital and
Royal National Hospital for Rheumatic Diseases,
Bath

Blackwell Scientific Publications
OXFORD LONDON
EDINBURGH BOSTON MELBOURNE

To Vanessa and Nicholas

© 1989 by
Blackwell Scientific Publications
Editorial offices:
Osney Mead, Oxford OX2 0EL
8 John Street, London WC1N 2ES
23 Ainslie Place, Edinburgh EH3 6AJ
3 Cambridge Center, Suite 208
 Cambridge, Massachusetts
 02142, USA
107 Barry Street, Carlton
 Victoria 3053, Australia

All rights reserved. No part of this
publication may be reproduced,
stored in a retrieval system, or
transmitted, in any form or by any
means, electronic, mechanical,
photocopying, recording or
otherwise without the prior
permission of the copyright owner

First published 1989

Set by Setrite Typesetters, Hong Kong,
and printed and bound
in Great Britain by
The Alden Press, Oxford

DISTRIBUTORS

Marston Book Services Ltd
PO Box 87
Oxford OX2 0DT
(*Orders*: Tel: (0865) 791155
          Fax: (0865) 791927
          Telex: 837515)

USA
Year Book Medical Publishers
200 North LaSalle Street
Chicago, Illinois 60601
(*Orders*: Tel: (312) 726−9733)

Canada
The C.V. Mosby Company
5240 Finch Avenue East
Scarborough, Ontario
(*Orders*: Tel: (416) 298−1588)

Australia
Blackwell Scientific Publications
(Australia) Pty Ltd
107 Barry Street
Carlton, Victoria 3053
(*Orders*: Tel: (03) 347−0300)

British Library
Cataloguing in Publication Data

Campion, G.V.
 Rheumatology
 1. Man. Joints. Arthritis &
 rheumatic diseases
 I. Title II. Dixon, Allan St J.
 (Allan St John) III. Series
 616.7′2

ISBN 0−632−01112−2

Contents

Preface, iv

Acknowledgements, v

List of abbreviations, vi

1 The clinical history and examination, 1

2 Investigation of rheumatic disease, 39

3 Imaging in the rheumatic diseases, 59

4 Regional problems and soft tissue rheumatism, 67

5 Important rheumatological conditions, 95

6 Therapy, 237

7 Skills in rheumatology, 277

Appendices, 297

Index, 309

Preface

This book is designed to give readily accessible and up-to-date information to all who look after patients suffering from arthritis and common bone diseases. Registrars and house officers, GPs, medical students and those in the paramedical professions should find here the guidance they need in the diagnosis, treatment and rehabilitation of their patients. This is not a text book, but a compact guide that can be carried around easily. Readers will still need to go to their libraries for in-depth knowledge and discussions on topics which in a small volume we have had to deal with somewhat dogmatically, guided by our practical experience. We have used UK spelling for words such as paediatric, orthopaedic, etc., to conform to the publisher's house style but the authors have worked extensively in the USA and hope that American readers, for whom this book should be equally suitable, will overlook this!

Acknowledgements

To Dr Iain Watt, Consultant Radiologist, for his great help with the radiograph illustrations and legends used in this book. To Drs Calvin Brown, Charles Hutton, Gunnar Anderson, Tony Woolf, Paul Dieppe and Peter Maddison for their help and advice regarding the material in various chapters. To the departments of Physiotherapy, Occupational Therapy and Social Work, the Royal National Hospital for Rheumatic Diseases, Bath, for help with Chapter 6, section 2.

To Eular Publishers for permission to publish illustrations for section 7.1 from A. St J. Dixon & J. Graber (1978) *Local Injection Therapy*; to Churchill Livingstone for permission to publish a modified version of Table 26.1, p. 483 as printed in P. A. Dieppe *et al.* (1985) *Rheumatological Medicine*; to W. B. Saunders for permission to publish a copy of Fig. 1 and Table 2 from H. A. Smythe (1979) Fibrositis as a Disorder of Pain Modulation. In *Clinics in Rheumatic Diseases* Vol. 5, No. 3. and to DIAL (Wiltshire) whose help is acknowledged in compiling Appendix 1. Also to Microsoft Word, Compaq and Hewlett Packard, without whom this work would not have been completed.

To Dr Michael Ahern of the Daw Park Hospital, Adelaide, for his work on the preliminary drafts of this book. Lastly, to Victoria Reeders from Blackwell Scientific Publications for her help and support during the project.

List of abbreviations

ACL	Anticardiolipin antibody
APTT	Activated partial thromboplastin time
ARC	Arthritis and Rheumatism Council
AS	Ankylosing spondylitis
CMI	Cell mediated immunity
CREST	Calcinosis, Raynaud's, oesophagitis, sclerodactyly, telangiectasia
CRP	C-reactive protein
CT	Computerized axial tomography
DIP	Distal interphalangeal (joint)
DM	Dermatomyositis
ESR	Erythrocyte sedimentation rate
GCA	Giant cell arteritis
HLA	Human lymphocyte antigen
IP	Interphalangeal (joint)
MCP	Metacarpophalangeal (joint)
MCTD	Mixed connective tissue disease
MRI	Magnetic resonance imaging
NSAID	Non-steroidal anti-inflammatory drug
OA	Osteoarthritis
PA	Pernicious anaemia
PAN	Polyarteritis nodosa
PIP	Proximal interphalangeal (joint)
PMR	Polymyalgia rheumatica
PTH	Parathyroid hormone
RA	Rheumatoid arthritis
RF	Rheumatoid factor
SIJ	Sacro-iliac (joint)
SLE	Systemic lupus erythematosus
SS	Systemic sclerosis
TB	Tuberculosis

1 The clinical history and examination

1.1 The clinical history, 3

1.2 The clinical examination, 19

1 The clinical history and examination

1.1 The clinical history

1.1 The clinical history

Diagnosis
The present classification of rheumatic disease is far from perfect. We are still ignorant about the aetiology and pathogenesis of many of the rheumatic diseases and many conditions are described mainly by clinical presentation. As a result, there is a large degree of overlap in the various 'separate conditions', with little information gained from the diagnosis about pathogenesis, disease process, prognosis and outcome. For the time being the approach to clinical diagnosis follows various broad guidelines.
- Is it primarily the joints or the soft tissues that are involved?
- Is it an inflammatory or mechanical process?
- What is the distribution of joint involvement?
- What is the disease course?
- Are extra-articular features present?
- What is the patient demography — age, sex, race?

The second guide to clinical diagnosis comprises the adages: common things occur commonly and rare complications of common diseases occur more commonly than rare diseases.

Disease impact
Rheumatology differs from some specialties in that many of the diseases are chronic and lead to varying degrees of disability. Therefore, it is vital to assess the impact of the disease on the patient's ability to lead a normal life.

Continuing care
Initial diagnosis forms only a small part of the physician's role. Follow-up of the patient involves:
1 Reassessment of diagnosis.
2 Monitoring response to therapy including possible adverse reactions.
3 Disease progression and complications.
4 Social aspects.

1 The clinical history and examination

1.1 The clinical history

The history

The age, sex and race of the patient. Reiter's syndrome and ankylosing spondylitis occur in young males. One would hesitate diagnosing them as presenting for the first time in an elderly female. On the other hand, polymyalgia rheumatica is a disease of the elderly and is unusual under 60 years. The age and sex of a patient may help in subtleties of diagnosis. Osteoarthritis developing in an elderly person is common and usually no underlying cause is found. Osteoarthritis occurring in a young person is unusual and would suggest an underlying cause (e.g. hip dysplasia or metabolic disease such as haemochromatosis or ochronosis).

Race. Some diseases are more prominent in people of different races: e.g. SLE in blacks, Behçet's syndrome in people of Eastern Mediterranean origin.

Inflammatory or mechanical. In practice some mixture often occurs. Inflammatory disease is characterized by:
  swelling;
  heat;
  pain;
  erythaema;
  loss of function;
  significant early morning stiffness;
  response to NSAID therapy.
Mechanical pain is:
  exacerbated by weight bearing;
  rapidly diminished by rest;
  sometimes accompanied by transient stiffness (less than 10 min duration).

1 The clinical history and examination

1.1 The clinical history

Distribution of joint involvement. This feature is often very helpful for diagnosis. Articular involvement may be:

monarticular	1 joint affected
oligoarticular	2–5 joints affected
polyarticular	>5 joints affected
asymmetrical or symmetrical	

Rheumatoid arthritis is characteristically a symmetrical, peripheral polyarthritis, with the brunt of the disease falling on the hands, wrists, knees and feet. Ankylosing spondylitis is predominantly an axial disease involving the sacro-iliac joints and spine. Reiter's syndrome is usually an asymmetrical oligoarthropathy affecting the lower limb joints (Table 1.1).

Disease course and progression. RA is a chronic disease with remissions and exacerbations, which usually leads to joint damage. The onset of viral arthritis caused by rubella or human parvovirus may closely resemble RA in the nature and distribution of joint involvement, but is self-limiting and does not cause chronic joint damage. A flitting arthritis may occur in gonococcal arthritis. A chronic insidious monarthritis is a typical feature of tuberculous arthritis.

Extra-articular features may be prominent in some rheumatic diseases. An inflammatory polyarthropathy such as RA may have a large systemic component: malaise, fatigue and weight loss. Associated features may include dry eyes and mouth (Sjögren's syndrome), subcutaneous nodules and rashes (vasculitis). Screening should include specific questions about:

General health	Malaise, fever, weight loss
The skin and scalp	Psoriasis, vasculitis, photosensitivity, gonorrhoea, alopecia
The gut	Mouth ulcers (Reiter's, SLE, Behçet's), dysphagia (SS), altered

1 The clinical history and examination

1.1 The clinical history

Table 1.1. Patterns of joint involvement in rheumatic disorders

1 *Causes of monoarthritis*
- (a) Septic arthritis including tuberculosis
- (b) Gout
- (c) Pseudogout
- (d) Trauma
- (e) Intra-articular loose body
- (f) Osteochondritis dissecans
- (g) Haemarthrosis
- (h) Erythema nodosum
- (i) Monarticular presentation of polyarticular disease
  Rheumatoid arthritis
  Seronegative spondyloarthropathies
  Chronic juvenile arthritis
- (j) Plant thorn synovitis
- (k) Neuropathic arthropathy
- (l) Avascular necrosis
- (m) Pigmented villonodular synovitis
- (n) Juxta-articular neoplastic tumours
- (o) Synovioma
- (p) Leukaemia, especially in children
- (q) Familial Mediterranean fever
- (r) Hyperlipoproteinaemias
- (s) Amyloid arthropathy

2 *Causes of oligoarthritis*
- (a) Osteoarthritis
- (b) Ankylosing spondylitis
- (c) Reiter's syndrome
- (d) Psoriatic arthropathy
- (e) Juvenile chronic arthritis
- (f) Sarcoid arthritis
- (g) Enteropathic arthritis
- (h) Behçet's syndrome
- (i) Septic arthritis
- (j) Pyrophosphate arthropathy
- (k) Gout
- (l) Familial Mediterranean fever
- (m) Hyperlipoproteinaemia

3 *Causes of polyarthritis*
- (a) Rheumatoid arthritis
- (b) Osteoarthritis (generalized nodal osteoarthritis)
- (c) Seronegative spondyloarthropathies
- (d) Systemic lupus erythematosus
- (e) Scleroderma
- (f) Sjögren's syndrome
- (g) Polyarteritis nodosa
- (h) Rheumatic fever
- (i) Viral arthritis
- (j) Septic arthritis, especially due to gonococcus
- (k) Dermatomyositis, polymyositis
- (l) Gout
- (m) Serum sickness

1 The clinical history and examination

1.1 The clinical history

	bowel habit, colitis (Crohn's, ulcerative colitis), dysentery (Reiter's), steatorrhoea (SS, Whipples)
Raynaud's	Systemic sclerosis, SLE, RA, dermatomyositis
The eyes	Dryness (Sjögren's), iritis (AS), conjunctivitis (Reiter's), scleritis (RA)
The urogenital tract	Dysuria, balanitis, cervicitis (Reiter's), ulceration (Behçet's)

Response to therapy. Most patients will have received some form of therapy prior to presentation. The effect of NSAIDs on inflammatory symptoms should be noted as well as any adverse effects. The response of PMR to adequate doses of steroids is prompt and dramatic and may itself be used as a diagnostic test (see section 5.6). Disease-remittive agents used in RA need to be monitored for efficacy and signs of toxicity. Some drugs may cause rheumatic symptoms in their own right, e.g. hydralazine can cause a lupus-like syndrome.

Past history. Some important aspects have been covered through specific questioning outlined above. The occurrence of arthritis in childhood should be enquired about. A previous history of TB may be valuable in an unexplained monarticular disease or may impose caution when instituting immunosuppressive therapy.

Family history of psoriasis, inflammatory bowel disease, ankylosing spondylitis or RA may aid diagnosis.

Social history. Enquire about the impact of disease on employment and on the activities of daily living such as:
   mobility, using taps, keys;
   toileting and personal hygiene;
   preparing and eating meals.
It is important to enquire whether the patient lives alone, and

1 The clinical history and examination

1.1 The clinical history

whether any form of occupational assessment has been performed.

Smoking is a general health problem, but may cause particular problems in patients with ankylosing spondylitis. Hypertrophic pulmonary osteoarthropathy arises secondary to bronchial carcinoma.

Occasionally *occupation* may be of relevance to disease diagnosis as with the occurrence of brucellosis in farmers and vets. Disease may also be modified by occupation, e.g. 'typus robustus' form of RA in manual workers.

Regional pain syndromes

Shoulder pain
See section 4.3.

Elbow pain
The elbow may be involved as part of a generalized polyarthropathy such as rheumatoid arthritis and seronegative spondyloarthropathies. It may become infected as in septic arthritis. Osteoid osteoma may involve the elbow especially in children and can simulate primary joint disease.

Pain may arise from the surrounding soft tissues as in lateral epicondylitis (tennis elbow), medial epicondylitis (golfer's elbow) and olecranon bursitis.

Hand and wrist pain
Pain in the hands and wrists may arise from numerous causes (Table 1.2).

Neck pain
Neck pain is a common source of complaint, but is usually less disabling than back pain. For a list of causes of neck pain see section 4.2. Enquire about:

1 The clinical history and examination

1.1 The clinical history

Table 1.2. Causes of pain in the hands and wrists

1 *Joints*
   (a) Inflammatory polyarthropathies, especially rheumatoid arthritis
   (b) Septic arthritis
   (c) Osteoarthritis

2 *Bones and periosteum*
   (a) Trauma such as fractures
   (b) Sarcoidosis
   (c) Hypertrophic pulmonary osteoarthropathy
   (d) Metastatic tumour, especially bronchogenic carcinoma

3 *Soft tissues*
   (a) Pulp or palmar space infection
   (b) Tenosynovitis, de Quervain's, flexor and extensor tendon sheaths, trigger finger
   (c) Paronychia
   (d) Subungual haematoma
   (e) Tendon rupture
   (f) Ganglion

4 *Referred pain — paraesthesiae*
   (a) Carpal tunnel syndrome
   (b) Ulnar nerve compression
   (c) Thoracic outlet syndrome
   (d) Shoulder hand syndrome
   (e) Brachial neuritis

Occupation and age. Acute neck strain and torticollis occur in younger people; cervical spondylosis occurs in older people. Symptoms may be exacerbated by any occupation requiring extremes of movement (e.g. painters and decorators).

Trauma. Ascertain the nature of the accident. If automobile accident, the type of collision, position of the patient in the vehicle. Is litigation impending?

Onset. Acute in acute neck strain, chronic in cervical spondylosis.

1 The clinical history and examination

1.1 The clinical history

Pain radiation. Pain from the upper cervical spine commonly radiates into the head and may be occipital, temporal, frontal and retro-orbital. Pain may also radiate to the shoulders, and upper limbs to the fingers.

Paraesthesia may indicate nerve involvement and can occur without demonstrable sensory loss.

Weakness will occur with involvement of the motor nerve fibres. Weakness of the legs may be the first sign of cord compression, especially in patients with rheumatoid involvement of the cervical spine.

Back pain (See also section 4.1)
Enquire about:
1 Age:
   (a) childhood (uncommon, usually clear cause)
   (b) young adult (acute ligamentous injury, disc prolapse, inflammatory disease such as ankylosing spondylitis)
   (c) middle-aged, elderly (facet joint arthritis, osteoporosis, spinal stenosis, metastatic disease).
2 Length of pain:
   (a) acute in intervertebral disc prolapse, ligamentous injury, osteoporotic collapse, trauma-related injury. In acute back strain, pain is generalized over the low back, accompanied by muscle spasm and moderate protective flexion
   (b) chronic in arthritis of the facet joint and with muscle fatigue.
3 Exacerbating and relieving factors:
   (a) exacerbated by sneezing, straining at stool (disc prolapse)
   (b) exacerbated by rest and relieved by exercise (inflammatory back disease)
   (c) exacerbated by exercise and relieved by rest (disc prolapse, spinal stenosis, facet joint arthritis).
4 Presence of prolonged morning stiffness:

1 The clinical history and examination

1.1 The clinical history

   (a) often prominent in inflammatory back disease, relieved by NSAIDs.
5 Neurological features:
   (a) paraesthesiae and weakness (disc prolapse). If present only on walking and relieved by rest suggestive of spinal cord stenosis bladder and bowel dysfunction (central disc prolapse or other cauda equina lesion).

The hip (Table 1.3)
Patients use the term 'hip' to describe not only the hip joint, but also the general region of the greater trochanter and side of the pelvis.

Pain arising in the hip joint is felt in the groin and may also be referred to the anterior thigh and knee, so that many with hip disease and a limp present as apparently having a knee problem.

Knee pain
Knee pain may arise from the knee joint, from surrounding structures or may be referred to the knee from the hip or lumbar spine (Table 1.4).

Foot and ankle pain
The ankle is a simple hinge joint allowing only plantar flexion and dorsiflexion. Ankle pain may arise from the joint itself or surrounding tissues such as tendon sheaths and the posterior subtaloid joint (Table 1.5).

System review
Many rheumatic diseases have systemic complications and conversely rheumatic symptoms may be secondary to disease elsewhere (e.g. thyroid disease). Elderly patients may have multiple pathology and the coexistence of heart failure due to ischaemic heart disease may be an important consideration when using NSAID therapy.

1 The clinical history and examination

1.1 The clinical history

Table 1.3. Causes of pain in the hip region

1 *Hip joint*
  (a) Chronic arthritis — OA, RA, ankylosing spondylitis
  (b) Aseptic necrosis
  (c) Septic arthritis including tuberculosis
  (d) Pigmented villonodular synovitis

2 *Acetabulum and femur*
  (a) Stress fractures, especially in osteomalacia
  (b) Primary or secondary tumours
  (c) Paget's disease

3 *Periarticular soft tissues*
  (a) Trochanteric bursitis
  (b) Bursa over the ischial tuberosity
  (c) Tendons and fascia
  (d) Hernia
  (e) Meralgia paraesthetica
  (f) Synovial cyst arising in the hip

4 *Referred pain*
  (a) Lumbosacral — facet joint OA
  (b) Nerve root irritation, e.g. prolapsed intervertebral disc
  (c) Viscera — kidneys, ureters
  (d) Femoral vein thrombophlebitis
  (e) Vascular insufficiency — Leriche syndrome (buttock claudication, impotence, absent femoral pulses)
  (f) Abscess in iliac fossa from appendicitis or diverticulitis
  (g) Psoas abscess from tuberculosis of the spine

Nervous system

Headaches
- Associated with muzziness may indicate sensitivity to NSAIDs such as indomethacin.
- In cervical spondylosis, pain is felt in the neck and occiput going through to behind the eyes.
- Felt superficially in the scalp, with pain on combing the hair suggests giant cell arteritis.

1 The clinical history and examination

1.1 The clinical history

Table 1.4. Causes of pain in the knee

1 *Pain arising in the knee region*
  (a) Femur — tumours, osteomyelitis, leukaemia
  (b) Prepatella bursa — bursitis
  (c) Collateral ligaments — sprain, osteoarthritis, Pellegrini — Stieda disease (calcification in the medial ligament)
  (d) Patella — patellofemoral osteoarthritis, chondromalacia patellae
  (e) Tibia — Osgood–Schlatter disease
  (f) Popliteal fossa — Baker's cyst, aneurysm
  (g) Fat pads — cold sensitive fat pads

2 *The knee joint*
  (a) Synovium — inflammatory arthritis, synovial rupture
  (b) Meniscus — tear
  (c) Loose body
  (d) Cruciate ligaments — trauma

3 *Referred pain*
  (a) Hip disease
  (b) Spine disease — L3 nerve root irritation

Table 1.5. Causes of foot and ankle pain

1 *Ankle pain*
  (a) Ankle joint
    Osteoarthritis
    Rheumatoid arthritis
    Seronegative spondylarthropathies
    Septic arthritis
    Aseptic necrosis
    Neuropathic arthritis
    Erythema nodosum arthritis (may precede skin changes)
  (b) Subtaloid joint
    Rheumatoid arthritis
  (c) Tendon sheaths
    Sports injuries
    Inflammatory arthropathies
  (d) Ligaments
    Trauma

1 The clinical history and examination

1.1 The clinical history

Table 1.5. (cont.)

2 *Heel pain*
- (a) Plantar fasciitis
- (b) Achilles tendinitis
- (c) Achilles bursitis
- (d) Ruptured achilles tendon
- (e) Rheumatoid nodules

3 *Foot pain*
- (a) Joints
  RA involving multiple joints — metatarsophalangeal joints (MTP)
  One or two joints — septic arthritis, seronegative spondyloarthropathies
  First MTP joint — as above as well as gout and hallux rigidus
- (b) Soft tissues
  Infection
- (c) Bones
  Stress fractures of metatarsals
  Osteochondritis of metatarsal heads (Freiberg's disease)
  Tumours
- (d) Nerves
  Neuroma of interdigital nerve
  Peripheral neuropathy
  Tarsal tunnel syndrome
  S1 irritation
- (e) Vessels
  Peripheral vascular disease
  Algodystrophy (Sudek's atrophy)

Visual problems
- Acute sudden loss of vision is a feared complication of giant cell arteritis.
- Cataracts can occur in long-term systemic steroid therapy.
- Maculopathy is associated with antimalarial treatment.

Numbness and tingling
- When localized may be due to nerve compression syndromes such as carpal tunnel syndrome or prolapsed intervertebral disc.

1 The clinical history and examination

1.1 The clinical history

- A glove and stocking peripheral neuropathy is a complication of various rheumatic diseases including rheumatoid arthritis and polyarteritis nodosa.
- Multiple peripheral nerves are involved in mononeuritis multiplex which is found in polyarteritis, rheumatoid arthritis, diabetes and leprosy.

Weakness
- Is common to most rheumatic diseases. If this presents as a sudden exacerbation in a patient with rheumatoid arthritis with neck involvement consider atlanto-axial subluxation with cord compression.
- Proximal weakness is prominent in inflammatory disease of muscle such as polymyositis and dermatomyositis. Consider also endocrinological and metabolic causes such as thyroid disease, Cushing's syndrome, acromegaly and osteomalacia.

Mood change
- Depression can lead to changes in sleep pattern associated with fibrositis. It may also be a systemic feature of SLE. Reactive depression may occur with chronic disability.

Major cerebrovascular events
- May be a presenting feature of SLE and the vasculitides.

Ear, nose and throat

'Saddle nose'
- Found in relapsing polychondritis, Wegener's granulomatosis and congenital syphilis.

Rhinitis
- Together with asthma is often prominent in Churg–Strauss vasculitis.

1 The clinical history and examination

1.1 The clinical history

Salivary gland swelling
- Sjögren's syndrome, sarcoidosis.

External ear
- Floppy, swollen pinnae from cartilage softening in the ears is characteristic of polychondritis.

Dryness of mouth and eyes
- Sjögren's syndrome.

Heart and lungs

Breathlessness
- Interstitial fibrosis in rheumatoid arthritis, systemic sclerosis and SLE.
- Apical fibrosis together with restricted chest wall movement may cause respiratory problems in ankylosing spondylitis.
- Pulmonary hypertension in CREST syndrome.
- Pericarditis can occur in all the systemic diseases of connective tissue. Constrictive pericarditis may develop insidiously in patients with long-standing rheumatoid arthritis.
- Valvular heart disease in seronegative spondyloarthropathies, rheumatoid arthritis, SLE and rheumatic fever.
- Cardiomyopathy in systemic sclerosis and amyloidosis.
- Anaemia of chronic disease and in chronic blood loss.

Pleuritic chest pain
- Serositis in rheumatoid arthritis and SLE.
- Chest wall myalgia in Bornholm disease.
- Enthesitis in ankylosing spondylitis.

Gastrointestinal

Mouth
- Inability to open the mouth widely (microstomia) in SS.

1 The clinical history and examination

1.1 The clinical history

- Build-up of pain in temporalis muscles (jaw claudication) in giant cell arteritis.

Ulcers
- Painful (penicillamine, gold, cytotoxic agents, Crohn's disease, SLE, Behçet's syndrome).
- Painless (Reiter's syndrome).

Dysphagia
- Painful mouth (ulcers, candidiasis).
- Poor salivation (Sjögren's syndrome).
- Dysmotility (systemic sclerosis).
- Mechanical (anterior exuberant cervical osteophytes).
- Oesophagitis (systemic sclerosis, NSAIDs, candidiasis).

Dyspepsia
- NSAIDs, corticosteroids.

Abdominal pain
- Peptic ulceration (NSAIDs, vasculitis).
- Mesenteric vasculitis (polyarteritis, Henoch–Schönlein purpura).
- Vascular thrombosis in SLE.
- Serositis may mimic an acute abdomen in SLE.
- Colitis.

Diarrhoea
- Colitis.
- Steatorrhoea, Whipple's disease, systemic sclerosis.
- Reiter's syndrome

Skin
Rashes give valuable clues in the following:
- Erythema marginatum, rheumatic fever.
- Henoch–Schönlein purpura (macular erythema with purpuric

1 The clinical history and examination

1.1 The clinical history

elements on the buttocks).
- Erythema nodosum arthritis (typical, blotchy, tender bruising with fixed lumps on the shins).
- Scattered 'rose spots' and small pustules in gonococcal arthritis.
- Erythema chronicum migrans, Lyme disease.

Numerous types of rash occur in sensitivity to drugs given for rheumatic conditions, ranging from a sheet-like erythema in phenylbutazone sensitivity to vasculitic changes and Stevens−Johnson syndrome.

Genito-urinary system

Dysuria
- Reiter's syndrome, gonorrhoea.

Ulcers
- Reiter's syndrome, Behçet's syndrome.

Balanitis
- Reiter's syndrome − may be best clue to diagnosis.

Nocturia
- May be first symptom of renal involvement in SLE.

Difficulty with urination
- Urgent symptom in cord compression.

1 The clinical history and examination

1.2 The clinical examination

1.2 The clinical examination

The examination begins as the patient enters the consulting room. Abnormalities of gait may indicate underlying joint pathology. Functional difficulties may become obvious as the patient attempts to undress or to climb on to the examination couch. The function of the examination is to enable the following questions to be answered.

- Can the diagnosis suggested by the history be confirmed?
- How active is the disease process?
- What functional problems are there?
- Is there any evidence of complications of the primary disease?
- Is any other pathology present?

There are several helpful points to remember in the examination of the musculoskeletal system.

- Adequate exposure of the affected part is essential.
- Weight-bearing joints should be examined with the patient upright and supine.
- Always examine the joints above and below the symptomatic one.
- Subtle changes in joints may be elicited if they are compared with the joint on the opposite side.

For practical purposes, screening procedures as indicated below are sufficient for the examination of range of motion of asymptomatic joints.

The hands and wrists

Inspect for swelling, muscle wasting or deformities, such as:

Swan-neck deformity: hyperextension of the PIP, flexion of DIP joint;

Boutonnière deformity: flexion of PIP, hyperextension of DIP joint;

Z-deformity of the thumb: flexion of metacarpal joint, hyperextended IP joint.

Palpate for increased warmth, localized tenderness and determine whether any swelling is soft or hard.

1 The clinical history and examination

1.2 The clinical examination

Range of movement

Screening
Ask the patient to flex the hands at the wrists, to oppose the palmar surfaces (as in praying), and then to elevate the elbows. Wrist inflammation will make the manoeuvre difficult and daylight between the fingers may indicate flexion deformities of the fingers.

Extension of the wrists can then be assessed by instructing the patient to oppose the dorsal aspects of the wrists and to lower the elbows.

The status of the finger joints can be assessed further by asking the patient to curl the fingers in as tightly as possible.

Measurement

Wrist
Extension: 70°; (C6,7) extensor carpi radialis longus and brevis, extensor carpi ulnaris (radial nerve).
Flexion: 80°; (C7,8) flexor carpi radialis (median), flexor carpi ulnaris (ulnar).
Ulnar deviation: 30°.
Radial deviation: 20°.

Hand
Finger extension: MCP joint 30°, PIP 0°, DIP 10°; (C7) extensors digitorum communis, indicis, digiti minimi (radial nerve).
Finger flexion: (C8)
  DIP joint (90°) flexor digitorum profundus (median);
  PIP joint (110°) flexor digitorum superficialis (median);
  MCP joint (90°) medial 2 lumbricals (ulnar), lateral 2 lumbricals (median).
Finger adduction: (T1) palmar interossei (ulnar).
Finger abduction: (T1) dorsal interossei, abductor digiti minimi (ulnar).

1 The clinical history and examination

1.2 The clinical examination

Thumb extension: MCP joint (50°) extensor pollicis brevis, IP joint (5°) extensor pollicis longus (radial nerve).

Thumb flexion: MCP joint (50°) flexor pollicis brevis (median and ulnar), IP joint (90°) flexor pollicis longus (median).

Thumb adduction: adductor pollicis (ulnar).

Thumb abduction: (70°) abductor pollicis brevis and longus (median).

Opposition of thumb and little finger: opponens pollicis (median), opponens digiti minimi (ulnar).

Test functional movements, grip, pinch grip. Test for carpal tunnel syndrome and digital vasculitis in RA and any complications of the disease. Run your hands up the extensor surface of the lower arms looking for subcutaneous nodules.

Special tests

Carpal tunnel syndrome

Tinel's test: percussion over the median nerve with the hand supinated.

Phalen's test: the patient should flex his wrists and hold them together for 60 sec. Both tests are positive if pain and/or paraesthesiae occur in the distribution of the median nerve.

de Quervain's tenosynovitis (stenosing tenosynovitis of abductor pollicis longus)

Finkelstein's test: the thumb is flexed across the palmar surface of the wrist and then a fist is made. The hand is then deviated to the ulnar side causing pain distal to the styloid process of the radius.

1 The clinical history and examination

1.2 The clinical examination

The elbows
These are often a rich source of clues in rheumatological diagnoses.

Inspect for deformity, swelling, subcutaneous nodules, psoriatic plaques. Nodules are found in rheumatoid arthritis, gout, xanthomatosis, calcinosis and rheumatic fever.

Palpate for increased heat and tenderness. Is tenderness localized to the joint line, or is it periarticular (e.g. the lateral epicondyle of the humerus in 'tennis elbow')?

Range of movement
Flexion: 135°; brachialis, biceps (with forearm supinated) (C5,6).
Extension: 0–5°; triceps (C7,8).
Supination: 90°; biceps, supinator.
Pronation: 90°; pronator teres, pronator quadratus.

Special tests

Lateral epicondylitis. In Cozen's test, the upper arm is stabilized by the examiner and with the lower arm flexed at 90°, resisted dorsiflexion is performed. In a positive test, pain is felt at the lateral epicondyle.

Medial epicondylitis. The patient is seated and asked to flex the elbow and supinate the hand. Pain over the medial epicondyle will occur with resisted elbow extension.

The shoulders
Inspect for swelling and deformity. Synovial effusion causes swelling anteriorly.

Palpate to localize pain. Pain may arise in any of the structures surrounding the shoulder.

1 Pain from the shoulder:
   (a) joints and bursae
       glenohumeral

1 The clinical history and examination

1.2 The clinical examination

      acromioclavicular
      subacromial bursa
  (b) muscles and tendons
      rotator cuff — supraspinatus. Pain is often referred to the lateral mid arm. Tenderness is maximal laterally, just inferior to the acromium
      rotator cuff — biceps: tendinitis gives pain anteriorly. The tendon may be palpated in the bicipital groove, 2.5 cm lateral to the coracoid process, with the upper arm externally rotated and the lower arm extended
  (c) 'trigger points' in fibrositis.

2 Referred pain — from the cervical spine.

In some cases it is possible to localize the problem from the clinical examination. In inflammatory arthropathies such as RA, a number of processes may be at work leading to a mixed picture.

Range of movement

Screening. Ask the patient to abduct both arms until above the head, to place both hands behind his head (external rotation) and to place the hand on the opposite scapula (internal rotation).

Measurement

Abduction: 180°; deltoid, supraspinatus (C5,6) will be impaired with supraspinatus rupture or tear.

Adduction: 45°; pectoralis major, latissimus dorsi (C6,7).

External rotation: 45°; keep the patient's elbow at his side and rotate the lower arm outwards. This is pure gleno-humeral movement and is achieved by the infraspinatus and teres minor muscles.

Internal rotation: 55°; subscapularis, pectoralis major.

Forward flexion: 90°; deltoid, coracobrachialis.

Extension: 50°; latissimus dorsi, teres major.

1 The clinical history and examination

1.2 The clinical examination

Movement is characteristically impaired in all directions in 'frozen shoulder' or adhesive capsulitis and in late rheumatoid arthritis.

Special tests

Rotator cuff

Painful arc. Ask the patient to elevate his arms fully and then to lower them slowly in abduction. Lesions affecting the rotator cuff or subacromial bursa will cause pain between 120° and 60° of abduction. If there is a rotator cuff tear, then the arm will drop to the side from about 90° (drop arm test).

Biceps

Yergason test. With the patient seated and elbow flexed to 90°, the examiner stabilizes the elbow and exerts lateral pressure against the patient's lower arm with resistance. Localized pain indicates tenosynovitis or instability of the biceps tendon.

The hip

Beware hip disease presenting as pain in the knee. Referred pain from the high lumbar spine may give thigh pain.

Initial observation of the patient will indicate hip disease.
1 The *antalgic gait*: patient spends as little time as possible weight-bearing on the painful hip.
2 Wasting of the buttock and thigh muscles.
3 Apparent leg length inequality due to adduction or abduction hip deformity.

Palpate for increased warmth and to localize pain. Typical hip pain is felt in the groin and radiates into the buttock. Tenderness is maximal anteriorly. If pain is atypical then with the patient supine, the following observations can be made:
- Tenderness medial to the anterior superior iliac spine with

1 The clinical history and examination

1.2 The clinical examination

numbness of the lateral hip and thigh suggests meralgia parasthetica.
- Examine the hernial orifices for incarcerated herniae, especially femoral.
- Tenderness of tendon insertions indicates tendon strain or enthesitis.

With the patient lateral, these observations are relevant:
- Tenderness over the lateral hip can indicate trochanteric bursitis.
- Tenderness over the ischial tuberosity occurs in ischial bursitis.

Leg length

The *apparent leg length* is measured from the xiphisternum to the medial malleolus on each side. Shortening is due to adduction contracture of the hip.

The *true length* is measured from the anterior superior iliac spine to the medial malleolus. Shortening is due to bony abnormality.

Range of movement

Compare both sides and use your other hand to fix the pelvis.

Rotation: internal 25°, external 35°. Pain in forced internal rotation often indicates the presence of a joint effusion.

Flexion: 120°; iliopsoas (L1).

Adduction: 25°; adductor longus (L2,3).

Abduction: 60°; gluteus medius (L5), the pelvis may be fixed conveniently by hanging the contralateral knee over the side of the couch.

Extension: 5–20°; gluteus maximus (S1).

Special tests

Weakness of hip abductors

The Trendelenburg sign. When the healthy subject stands on one leg, contraction of the contralateral hip abductors elevates the pelvis. In hip or neuromuscular disease the abductors are weakened and the contralateral pelvis falls.

Flexion deformity

Thomas's test. The patient lies supine on the couch and lumbar lordosis is eliminated by flexion of the good hip. If the contralateral hip rises from the couch then a fixed flexion deformity of that hip is present.

Shortening

The Allis test. The patient is supine, with the pelvis square and is asked to flex his hips so that both feet are resting on the couch at the same level. The height of the knees should be equal. If the affected side is lower, this indicates either posterior displacement of the femoral head or shortening of the femur or tibia.

The knee
1 With the patient erect *inspect* the knee weight bearing for any valgus or varus deformity.
2 With the patient supine *examine* the knees for contractures, scars or signs of trauma. A knee effusion is usually visible as loss of the small hollows which occur at each side of the patella. Loss of quadriceps bulk is common with knee pathology.
  Palpate for increased surface temperature.

Localized tenderness. Common sites include:
1 The medial and lateral joint line (easiest to examine with the knee flexed).
2 The patellofemoral joint (rock the patella from side to side with the knee extended).
3 The attachments of the medial and lateral collateral ligaments.

1 The clinical history and examination

1.2 The clinical examination

4 The bursae: pre-patella, superficial and deep infrapatella and anserine, (located between hamstring insertion and upper medial aspect of tibia, medial to the tibial tubercle).

5 The attachment of the patella tendon to the tibial tubercle may be tender in young people with Osgood−Schlatter syndrome.

Test for the presence of an effusion. Trace amounts of fluid can be detected by the fluid displacement test: one side of the knee is stroked upwards to remove fluid from that region, the other side is quickly stroked upwards and fluid flicks across below the patella.

Larger amounts of fluid give a positive patella tap, but it is generally obvious on inspection of the knee that an effusion is present.

Feel and inspect the back of the knee for a popliteal cyst (Baker's cyst).

Range of movement

Flexion: 135°; hamstrings (L5,S1), feel for joint crepitus.
Extension: 0−5°; quadriceps (L3,4), lift the leg whilst pressing down on the patella.

Stress the ligaments

Collateral. The easiest way to do this is by first stabilizing the knee to be tested by resting it on the contralateral knee. Then by further stabilizing the joint by one hand stress it medially and laterally.

Cruciate. Flex the knee to 90° and rest the patient's foot on the couch. Then try to displace the lower leg forwards (the anterior drawer test for anterior cruciate stability) and backwards (the posterior drawer test for posterior cruciate stability).

Remember pain originating from the hip may be felt in the knee.

1 The clinical history and examination

1.2 The clinical examination

The foot and ankle

Examine initially with the patient weight bearing.

Valgus deformity of the subtaloid joint is one of the commonest problems in rheumatoid arthritis and may be missed if the patient is examined only on the couch.

Examine for foot posture, medial and lateral arches.

Inspect, with the patient supine, for the following signs:

1 Ankle swelling, tendon sheath swelling, deformity of the forefoot including hallux valgus.

2 Synovitis of the metatarsal joints gives rise to the 'daylight sign', with visible spaces between the toes.

3 Examine the nails for signs of psoriatic involvement, check the soles for rashes such as keratoderma blenorrhagica associated with Reiter's syndrome.

Palpate for the following signs:

1 Increased warmth and localized tenderness.

2 Erythema and scaling over a tender 1st MTP joint is very suggestive of gout.

3 Feel for prominance and tenderness of the metatarsal heads with ulceration in RA.

4 Localized tenderness usually between the 3rd and 4th metatarsal head occurs with a plantar digital neuroma (Morton's metatarsalgia).

5 Tenderness under the calcaneum occurs in plantar fasciitis and with calcaneal spurs. Swelling of the achilles tendon in tendinitis may be more obvious when viewed posteriorly with the patient prone.

6 Stress fractures at the lower end of the fibula are not uncommon in arthritis patients. They can be confused with arthritis in the ankle. Test by gently rolling a pencil down the fibula towards the lateral malleolus. A sharply localized area of tenderness will be found if a stress fracture is present.

7 Pain over the posterior tibial nerve at the medial malleolus may occur in the tarsal tunnel syndrome. Test for paraesthesia in

1 The clinical history and examination

1.2 The clinical examination

the foot on percussion of the nerve and sensory changes in the sole of the foot.

8 Check the pedal pulses: dorsalis pedis and posterior tibial.

Range of movement

Ankle dorsiflexion: 15°; tibialis anterior, extensor hallucis longus, extensor digitorum longus (L4,5).

Plantar flexion: 55° (measured from the neutral position with the foot at 90° to the leg); gastrocnemius, soleus, peroneus longus and brevis (S1,2).

Inversion: 35°; tibialis anterior (L4,5).

Eversion: 20°; mainly occurs through the subtaloid joint, but also the mid-tarsal and tarso-metatarsal joints; peroneus longus and brevis (S1).

Tenosynovitis of the ankle tendons

1 *Tibialis posterior* rupture is a common cause of flat foot in RA. Look for tendon sheath swelling medially and pain on plantar flexion and eversion of the foot. The tendon may be tender or discontinuous (if ruptured).

2 *Peroneal tendons*. Tenderness and swelling laterally with pain on plantar flexion and inversion.

Stability of the ankle is provided by the medial (deltoid) and lateral (anterior and posterior talofibular and calcaneofibular) ligaments.

The anterior talofibular ligament is the most commonly involved ligament in sprains. Stress the ligament by plantar flexion and inversion, check for stability by pulling the hindfoot forwards whilst pushing back on the tibia (anterior draw sign).

Invert the hindfoot to check for lateral instability and evert for medial instability.

1 The clinical history and examination

1.2 The clinical examination

The spine and pelvis
Inspect the spine from the side looking for the normal thoracic kyphosis and lumbar lordosis.

Thoracic kyphosis	Increased in osteoporosis Angulated (gibbus) in TB of the spine, fractures and congenital vertebral abnormality
Lumbar lordosis	Diminished in ankylosing spondylitis, prolapsed intervertebral disc Increased as a normal variant, in spondylolisthesis, secondary to flexion deformity of the hips
Scoliosis	A structural scoliosis can be distinguished from a functional scoliosis (e.g. due to prolapsed intervertebral disc) by observing the patient bending. With structural scoliosis the scoliosis will remain on bending whereas with functional scoliosis the deformity will disappear or the patient will be unable to bend due to pain
The skin	Scars, café au lait spots, skin tags Malignancy in AS patients treated by deep X-ray therapy

Palpate for localized tenderness in the following areas:
1 Vertebral spinous process (if marked) suggests infection or bony metastases of the vertebral body.
2 Between lumbar vertebral spines and the lumbosacral junction found in prolapsed disc.
3 Paraspinal muscles in low back strain and prolapsed disc;
4 Sacro-iliac joints, which may also be demonstrated by pain on stressing the joint in the pelvic rock test. In this, the patient lies

1 The clinical history and examination

1.2 The clinical examination

on his side and the examiner presses down hard on the ilium. This is repeated on the other side.

5 Do not forget intra-abdominal causes for back pain and test for tenderness in the renal angle.

Range of movement

Cervical spine

Anterior flexion: the patient should be able to put his chin on his chest.

Lateral flexion: to right and left 30°.

Extension: 30°; the patient should be able to look at the ceiling.

Rotation: to left and right 80°; a spatula held in the patient's mouth may help as a pointer — the chin should end up almost in line with the shoulder.

Thoraco-lumbar spine and chest wall

Chest expansion: male = 5 cm, female = 4 cm.

Anterior flexion: ask the patient to touch his toes with the knees straight. The movement is a combination of spine and hip flexion. For an assessment of spinal mobility on flexion see the Schobers test below.

Lateral flexion: 30°; ask the patient to slide his hands down the thigh to the knee.

Extension: 30°; increased back pain upon extension in spondylolisthesis.

Rotation: 40°; measured between the plane of the shoulders and the spine. Stand behind the patient and stabilize the pelvis with one hand, then rotate by pulling on the opposite shoulder.

Special tests

Thoracic outlet syndrome

The Adson test. The radial pulse is palpated and the patient

1 The clinical history and examination

1.2 The clinical examination

instructed to make a maximal, held inspiration, with the head turned towards the affected side. The sign is positive if there is reduction in the radial pulse on the affected side and/or paraesthesiae in the upper extremity.

Cervical radiculopathy

The shoulder depression test is positive if reproduction of the symptoms occurs with depression of the shoulder and lateral flexion of the neck to the opposite side. A full neurological examination should be performed, looking for signs both in the upper limbs (usually lower motor neurone, see Table 1.6 and Fig. 1.1) and lower limbs (upper motor neurone).

Lumbar spine mobility

Schober's test. The patient should stand erect. Note the position of the spinous process of L5 (at the level of the 'dimples of Venus') and points 5 cm below and 10 cm above in the midline. The patient should then maximally bend forward, knees straight. The distance between the two points should increase by 5 cm or more; 4 cm or less indicates reduced mobility.

Prolapsed intervertebral disc
1 *Straight leg raising.* The patient is supine on the couch. Support the heel with one hand and place the other over the knee to keep the leg straight. Note the angle the leg may be raised before pain. Pain in the posterior thigh suggests tight hamstring muscles. Pain in the back or along the course of the sciatic nerve will occur in disc prolapse and will be exacerbated by passive dorsiflexion of the foot.
2 *Cross leg/straight leg raising test.* This is positive if the patient complains of back or sciatic pain on the involved side if the contralateral leg is raised.

1 The clinical history and examination

1.2 The clinical examination

3 *Reverse Lasegue test* stretches the femoral nerve roots and is performed if a high lumbar disc is suspected. The patient is prone and each knee is flexed in turn. Pain coming from a disc will be exacerbated by extension of the hip.

In a difficult patient, confirmation may be sought by instructing the patient to sit up on the couch. A patient with a low lumbar disc lesion will be unable to do so without flexing the knees. A disc lesion may be ruled out if the supine patient can hold both legs 5 cm above the couch for 30 sec (*Milgram test*). *Lindner's sign* is positive if neck flexion in the supine position reproduces the patient's sciatic pain.

Neurological examination of the legs should be performed (see Table 1.7 and Fig. 1.1).

In spinal stenosis, neurological signs may only become apparent after exercising the patient, or may not exist at all.

Hypermobility

There is an increased frequency of OA in patients with hypermobility. It is also associated with various inherited

Table 1.6. Effects of cervical nerve root compression. With disc prolapse it is the nerve root below the disc (most commonly C5/6) that is usually affected. Multiple lesions may occur

Nerve root	Muscle weakness	Reflexes	Sensation
C5	Deltoid Biceps	Biceps	Lateral upper arm
C6	Biceps Wrist extensors	Biceps	Lateral forearm, thumb, index finger
C7	Triceps Wrist flexors Finger extensors	Triceps	Middle finger
C8	Finger flexors	No change	Medial forearm, medial two fingers
T1	Finger abductors	No change	Medial upper arm

1 The clinical history and examination

1.2 The clinical examination

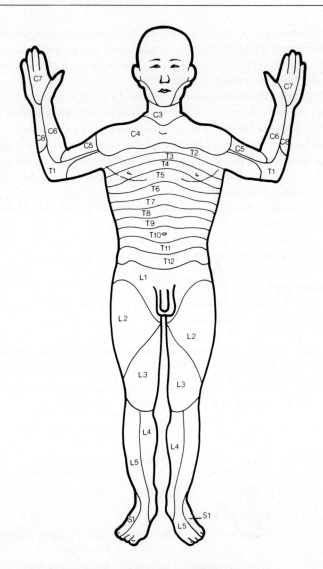

Fig. 1.1a Neurological dermatomes — anterior view.

1 The clinical history and examination

1.2 The clinical examination

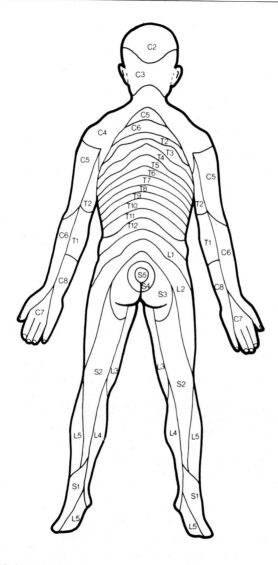

Fig. 1.1b Neurological dermatomes — posterior view.

1 The clinical history and examination

1.2 The clinical examination

Table 1.7. Effects of lumbar nerve root compression. L5 and S1 are the commonest nerve roots involved

Nerve root	Muscle weakness	Reflexes	Sensation
L2	Hip flexors and adductors	No change	Anterior upper thigh
L3	Hip adduction Knee extension Thigh wasting	Weak knee jerk	Anterior thigh to knee
L4	Hip extension and abduction Extension of knee Inversion of foot	Weak or absent knee jerk	Medial side of leg
L5	Extension of big toe Ankle dorsiflexion Calf wasting	No change	Lateral calf Dorsum of foot
S1	Plantar flexion Hip extension	Weak or absent ankle jerk	Lateral foot and sole

Table 1.8. Beighton scoring system for hyperlaxity

1 Passive dorsification of the little fingers over 90° (one point for each side)
2 Passive apposition of the thumb to the flexor part of the forearm (one point for each side)
3 Hyperextension of the elbows over 10° (one point for each side)
4 Hyperextension of the knees over 10° (one point for each side)
5 Forward flexion of the trunk with the kees straight, with the palms resting easily on the floor (one point)

disorders of connective tissue (see section 5.12). The Beighton scoring system (Table 1.8) is most frequently used for quantification of joint hyperlaxity. A high degree of laxity is suggested by a score of 6/9 points below the age of 40 and 4/9 over 40 years.

1 The clinical history and examination

1.2 The clinical examination

Schirmer's test

This is an easily administered bedside test for the detection of reduced tear secretion associated with primary or secondary Sjögren's syndrome (section 5.4). The test strips of filter paper are commercially available.

1 The patient should be comfortable and the procedure explained.

2 The patient is then requested to look up and the filter paper is folded slightly so as to hook over the lower eyelid.

3 The patient is then instructed to close the eyes.

4 Less than 5 mm wetting of the filter paper after 5 min indicates impaired tear secretion.

Capillaroscopy

Nailfold capillary loops are often abnormal in various connective tissue diseases. They may be examined in the outpatient clinic or at the bedside with an ophthalmoscope or other suitable magnifying equipment. A drop of oil is placed over the capillary bed for better resolution.

Capillary loops may not be visible in pigmented individuals. The ring and little finger have the longest capillaries and the most visible subpapillary plexus.

The technique appears to be most useful in systemic sclerosis and dermatomyositis. Changes include:

1 Widening of capillary loops.

2 Loss of loops in some areas.

3 Distorted bushy areas.

2 Investigation of rheumatic disease

2.1 Laboratory tests, 41

2.2 Other biochemical and haematological tests, 51

2 Investigation of rheumatic disease

2.1 Laboratory tests

2.1 Laboratory tests

Introduction

Laboratory tests perform a range of functions in the diagnosis and treatment of rheumatic diseases. They should be interpreted in the context of a careful history and physical examination. Laboratory tests are useful:

1 In differential diagnosis.
2 To exclude certain diseases.
3 To determine disease activity.
4 To monitor the effects of treatment.

Laboratory values that conflict with the clinical diagnosis should always be regarded with suspicion.

Acute phase reactants

Erythrocyte sedimentation rate (ESR)

The ESR is a measure of the rate of fall in mm per hour of anticoagulated red blood cells in a standard glass tube (Westergren method).

In inflammatory states, erythrocytes form stacks (rouleaux), that result from increased amounts of fibrinogen and which allow them to sediment more rapidly. A normal ESR tends to exclude active inflammatory states such as:

acute rheumatic fever;
systemic lupus erythematosis;
rheumatoid arthritis;
polymyalgia rheumatica.

The ESR is useful in monitoring disease course and response to medication.

Falsely low ESRs are found in:

1 Sickle cell disease.
2 Anisocytosis.
3 Spherocytosis.
4 Polycythaemia.

2 Investigation of rheumatic disease

2.1 Laboratory tests

5 Cardiac and hepatic failure.

The ESR has many limitations and measurement of plasma viscosity is the preferred investigation (Table 2.1).

Plasma viscosity

The plasma viscosity correlates highly with the ESR. Its major advantage over the ESR is that measurement can be automated and therefore it provides a simpler screening test for those abnormalities detected by the ESR.

It reflects the concentration of large molecular weight proteins, mainly fibrinogen, but also the abnormal immunoglobulins in multiple myeloma and macroglobulinaemia. Other advantages of plasma viscosity over ESR are listed in Table 2.1.

C-reactive protein (CRP)

CRP is an acute phase reactant protein synthesized by hepatocytes. Its rate of synthesis increases within hours of acute injury or the onset of inflammation (see Table 2.2). It may be measured by radial immunodiffusion, radioimmunoassay or laser nephelometry.

Measurement of CRP in clinical practice may be valuable in:
1 The management and assessment of disease activity in such inflammatory states as RA, juvenile chronic arthritis, ankylosing

Table 2.1. Advantages of plasma viscosity over ESR

---

1 Independent of age and sex
2 Independent of smoking habits
3 Well defined narrow normal range
4 Very good reproducibility between different laboratories and within the same laboratory (coefficient of variation 1%)
5 Can keep the plasma sample up to 4 days at room temperature before analysis (4 hours with ESR)
6 Result obtained in 10 min
7 Independent of haemaglobin
8 Low incidence of false negatives
9 Little effect of circadian rhythms

2   Investigation of rheumatic disease

2.1   Laboratory tests

spondylitis, Reiter's syndrome, Crohn's disease and vasculitic illnesses.

2 Diagnosis and management of infection.

3 Differential diagnosis (e.g. SLE versus RA, and Crohn's disease versus ulcerative colitis).

In some inflammatory states, there may be an elevation of the ESR and white cell count with only a modest or absent CRP response. Examples include:

SLE;

dermatomyositis;

systemic sclerosis;

ulcerative colitis.

The CRP response is not directly affected by non-steroidal anti-inflammatory drugs or immunosuppressive drugs including steroids unless they affect the activity of the underlying disease process.

Rheumatoid factors

Rheumatoid factors are autoantibodies directed against antigenic determinants on the FC fragment of immunoglobulin G (IgG). Three immunoglobulin classes (IgM, IgA and IgG) have rheumatoid factor (RF) activity, but standard serological tests detect only IgM rheumatoid factors.

Sites of synthesis of RF are peripheral blood, bone marrow, synovium, lymph nodes and subcutaneous nodules. The stimulus for production of RF is unknown.

IgM rheumatoid factor

IgM rheumatoid factor is detected by agglutination reactions because of the pentavalent binding sites of IgM.

Latex test. Agglutination of IgG coated latex particles is the method most laboratories use. The quantity of IgM RF is then expressed as the highest dilution of serum yielding detectable agglutination.

2 Investigation of rheumatic disease

2.1 Laboratory tests

Rose–Waaler reaction. Red cells coated with human or rabbit IgG are also agglutinated by IgM RF.

Rheumatoid factor may be detected in 1–5% of the background population, its frequency rising with age, also in patients with diseases other than rheumatoid arthritis (Table 2.2).

Table 2.2. Conditions associated with a positive test for rheumatoid factor

Connective tissue diseases
  Rheumatoid arthritis with nodules 100%
  Rheumatoid arthritis without nodules 80%
  Sjögren's syndrome 80%
  Scleroderma 30%
  Systemic lupus erythematosus 30%

Acute viral conditions } 30%
  Epstein–Barr virus infection
  Hepatitis
  Influenza

Parasites } 30%
  Trypanosomiasis
  Leishmaniasis
  Malaria
  Schistosomiasis
  Filariasis

Chronic bacterial infections
  Infective endocarditis
  Tuberculosis
  Leprosy
  Yaws
  Syphilis
  Brucellosis
  Salmonella

Neoplasms

Other
  Sarcoid
  Chronic liver disease
  Fibrosing alveolitis
  Silicosis

2 Investigation of rheumatic disease

2.1 Laboratory tests

IgG rheumatoid factor
These are inefficient agglutinators of IgG coated particles or red blood cells and are usually detected by their sedimentation profile in the analytical ultracentrifuge. Three systemic complications of RA have been associated with IgG RFs:
  hyperviscosity syndrome;
  Felty's syndrome;
  rheumatoid vasculitis.

Antinuclear antibodies (ANA)
A wide range of antibodies to nuclear and cytoplasmic cellular antigens is found in various rheumatic diseases, particularly SLE. They are demonstrated by immunofluorescence, radioimmunoassay and immunodiffusion.

Indirect immunofluorescence
The immunofluorescent technique uses a cellular substrate (usually thin sections of frozen rat liver or kidney). Test sera diluted 1:10 or greater are added to the tissue sections, incubated and then washed.

Fluoroscein-labelled antibodies reactive with all immunoglobulins or class-specific for IgG, IgM or IgA are then layered over the sections. Immunofluorescent microscopy detects the presence of antibodies in the sera bound to nuclear components.

A variety of patterns representing antibodies to different cellular antigens can be detected (Table 2.3).

Certain nuclear and nucleolar antigens are absent in organs such as rodent liver and kidney and are present in rapidly proliferating tissue culture lines. This is important for detection of antibodies to Ro, anti-centromere antibody and RANA. RANA is a nuclear antigen derived from an EB virus infected cell line.

Anti-DNA antibodies
These can be classified into two types:

2 Investigation of rheumatic disease

2.1 Laboratory tests

1 Antibody recognizing an antigenic determinant common to both native (double stranded) and denatured (single stranded) DNA.
2 Antibody reacting with single stranded DNA only. These react with purine and pyrimidine bases which are hidden in native DNA.

Assays used for the detection of anti-DNA antibodies are:
1 Radioimmunoassay (Farr method).
2 *Crithidia luciliae* as substrate in indirect immunofluorescence.

In *clinical use*:
anti-double-stranded DNA antibody is present in high frequency (50–69%) and in high titres in SLE. High titres are often accompanied by low serum complement and active glomerulonephritis;
anti-single-stranded DNA antibody are present in various disease states, including drug-induced SLE and liver disease.

Antinuclear ribonucleoprotein (nRNP) antibodies
These are present in high titres in mixed connective tissue disease (MCTD) and are also present in SLE, scleroderma and discoid LE.

Serologically, patients with MCTD can be defined as having high titres of antibodies to nRNP. Whether such a group of patients with these serological criteria has distinct clinical features is debatable.

Antibodies to other nuclear constituents
See Table 2.3.

Other autoantibodies

Anticardiolipin antibody (ACL)
Circulating anticardiolipin antibody is responsible for the false positive screening tests for syphilis seen in some patients with SLE. It interferes with the binding of phospholipid to form

2 Investigation of rheumatic disease

2.1 Laboratory tests

Table 2.3. Immunospecificities of antinuclear antibodies

Immunospecificity	Disease association
1 Antibodies to DNA	
(a) Identical determinants on native and denatured DNA	High titres in SLE
(b) single stranded DNA	Present in rheumatic and non-rheumatic disease
2 Antibodies to histones	Occur in 30% of SLE; in 95% of procainamide-induced SLE
3 Antibodies to non-histone antigens	
(a) Sm antigen	Specific for SLE; occurs in 25% of patients with SLE
(b) Nuclear RNP	Present in high titres in MCTD
(c) Ro (SSA) and La (SSB)	High frequency in Sjögren's syndrome, occurs in 40% (Ro) and 20% (La) in SLE; present in 60% with subacute cutaneous LE
	Ro invariable in neonatal lupus, present in 60% of ANA negative SLE
(d) Scl-70	25% of scleroderma patients (highly specific)
(e) Centromere protein	Present in 90% of CREST variant of scleroderma
(f) RANA	RA, RANA is a nuclear antigen derived from an EB virus infected cell line
(g) Jo-1	Directed against histidyl-tRNA synthetase, present in 30% idiopathic polymyositis
(h) Mi	Polymyositis
(j) Ku	Polymyositis–scleroderma overlap
4 Antibodies to nucleolar antigens PM-Scl	Polymyositis–scleroderma overlap

2 Investigation of rheumatic disease

2.1 Laboratory tests

prothrombin activator and leads to a slight prolongation of the activated partial thromboplastin time (lupus anticoagulant).

Parodoxically, it has been reported to be found with increased frequency in patients with SLE and thrombosis, as well as pulmonary hypertension, autoimmune thrombocytopenia, temporal arteritis and Behçet's disease. It may also occur in patients with connective tissue disorders without these complications however. It is associated with recurrent miscarriage due to placental vein thrombosis with or without rheumatic symptoms.

Antibodies to neutrophil alkaline phosphatase
These have been reported in most patients with Wegener's granulomatosis and microscopic polyarteritis, and seem to correlate better with disease activity than other commonly used markers.

Complement
Serial measurements of complement levels may be helpful in guiding therapy in patients with SLE.

Quantification of complement or its components can be performed by haemolytic assays or by immunodiffusion using antisera specific for individual components.

Total haemolytic complement (CH50) is measured in haemolytic units and is an assay of the ability of the test serum to lyse 50% of a standard suspension of sheep red blood cells coated with rabbit antibody.

Complement deficiency states
- Deficiencies of early classical pathway components (especially C2) are associated with SLE-like syndromes and an increased susceptibility to infections.
- Deficiency of C1q esterase inhibitor is associated with hereditary angioedema.

2 Investigation of rheumatic disease

2.1 Laboratory tests

- Deficiency of C3b esterase inactivator creates an increased liability to infection.

Interpretation of complement levels
CH50 levels are often low in SLE, cryoglobulinaemia and systemic vasculitis as a consequence of circulating or fixed immune complexes.

Serum complement levels may be increased in RA, gout and the spondyloarthropathies as a result of being 'acute phase' reactants.

Immune complex assays
Current assays frequently correlate poorly with disease activity and are inappropriate for routine clinical application.

Cryoglobulins
Measurement of cryoglobulins is the simplest test for immune complexes; it is based on their decreased solubility at 4°C, with the formation of a cryoprecipitate.

They are found in diseases associated with immune complexes — SLE, rheumatoid vasculitis and essential cryoglobulinaemia. Sera with very large quantities of cryoglobulin nearly always contain monoclonal immuno-globulins.

The syringe should be preheated to 37°C before blood is drawn and the blood should be allowed to clot at 37°C. (The best way of doing this is to warm the blood tube and syringe in a thermos flask of water that has been kept in an incubator at 37°C. The blood should be placed into the warmed tube and then into the thermos flask and taken straight to the incubator.) Serum is separated at room temperature and an aliquot examined for precipitates after 2 days at 4°C.

2 Investigation of rheumatic disease

2.1 Laboratory tests

Biochemical tests

Serum uric acid
An elevated serum uric acid level does not diagnose gout. It may be elevated in obesity, hypothyroidism, hyperparathyroidism, renal failure, psoriasis and by drug therapy such as thiazide diuretics (see Table 5.3).

Plasma proteins
Inflammatory states will often show a reduction in serum albumin and a rise in gamma globulin. The gamma globulin level correlates with disease activity and may be very high in SLE.

Serum alkaline phosphatase
This is increased in both liver and bone disease. The origin of alkaline phosphatase can be determined by heat lability, isoenzyme separation or measurement of other liver enzymes such as gamma glutamyltransferase or 5-nucleotidase.

The common bone diseases causing an elevated serum alkaline phosphatase include:
fractures;
Paget's disease;
hyperparathyroidism;
osteomalacia;
bone tumours.
Very high levels indicate hepatic disease or Paget's disease.

Muscle enzymes
The serum creatinine phosphokinase (CPK) and serum aldolase are helpful in the diagnosis of dermatomyositis or polymyositis and in the monitoring of their response to therapy.

2.2 Other biochemical and haematological tests

For normal values and perturbations commonly associated with rheumatic disease see Table 2.4.

Synovial fluid (SF)
Examination of the synovial fluid can yield specific diagnoses such as crystal-induced arthritis and joint infection and may be helpful in the diagnosis of other arthropathies (see Table 2.4).

Gross examination

Colour
- Normal synovial fluid is colourless or a pale straw colour.
- Inflammatory fluids are yellow to green-yellow.
- Haemarthroses occur with:
    bleeding disorders;
    trauma (including trauma complicating OA or RA);
    neoplasms (especially villonodular synovitis);
    acute crystal synovitis (occasionally).
- Infected joint fluid resembles pus.

Clarity
Normal synovial fluid is clear and print can be read through it.

Viscosity
Synovial fluid viscosity is tested by allowing a drop of fluid to fall from the needle tip. Normal fluids are viscous and a viscous thread will form. Another impression of viscosity can be obtained if the syringe is shaken to produce bubbles. If the bubbles rise slowly the fluid is highly viscous. Inflammatory fluids have a decreased viscosity so no viscous thread is found and the bubbles rise quickly.

Cell count
This is performed on a counting chamber such as a haemocytometer. In normal fluid only a few cells are present.

Table 2.4. Normal laboratory values (may vary from laboratory to laboratory)

	Normal range		Notes
	Male	Female	
Haematology			
Hb	13.5–17.0 g/dl	11.5–15.5 g/dl	Anaemia of chronic disease common in active disease. Normocytic normo/hypochromic picture. Coombs positive haemolytic anaemia in SLE
Red cell vol.	30±5 ml/kg	25±5 ml/kg	
MCV	75–95 FL		
MCH	26–32 PG		
MCHC	31–35 g/dl		
Platelets	150–450 × 10^9/l		Low platelets, low WCC in Evan's syndrome found in SLE and drug toxicity
WCC	4–11 × 10^9/l		
Neutrophils	2.0–7.5 × 10^9/l		Neutropenia in Felty's syndrome
Eosinophils	0.04–0.4 × 10^9/l		Neutrophilia in PAN
Lymphocytes	1.5–4.0 × 10^9/l		Lymphopenia in SLE
Monocytes	0.2–0.8 × 10^9/l		Eosinophilia in Churg–Strauss, eosinophilic fasciitis
Reticulocytes	10–100 × 10^9/l (<2%)		
Viscosity	1.5–1.72 cp		
ESR, age	20–50 < 15 mm/h–< 25 mm/h		
	> 50 < 20 mm/h–< 30 mm/h		
Serology			
Se ferritin	16–330 ng/ml	4–120 ng/ml (premenopausal)	Best test for Fe deficiency when low; raised as part of the acute phase response
		12–230 ng/ml (postmenopausal)	

Se B$_{12}$	200–900 ng/l	
Se folate	3–20 mg/l	
Red cell folate	170–640 mg/l	
HbA$_2$	2–3.5%	
HbF	<1%	
Haptoglobins	20–200 mg/100 ml	Low in haemolytic anaemia; raised as part of the acute phase response

Biochemistry – blood

Bicarbonate	22–28 mmol/l	
Chloride	98–108 mmol/l	
Creatinine	53–150 mmol/l	
K	3.0–5.5 mmol/l	
Na	136–145 mmol/l	
Urea	2.5–6.6 mmol/l	
Bilirubin	3–20 mmol/l	
Aspartate amino transferase	5–35 IU/l	
Alkaline phosphatase	30–300 IU/l	Raised as part of the acute phase response, also osteomalacia, liver disease and Paget's
Calcium	2.1–2.6 mmol/l	Usually corrected for serum albumin: add 0.2 g/l for every g below 42 g/l
Phosphate	0.8–1.4 mmol/l	
Uric acid	0.20–0.42 mmol/l	0.15–0.36 mmol/l
Ascorbic acid	34–114 μmol/l	
C reactive protein	0–20 g/l	Useful indicator of the acute phase response
Albumin	39–45 g/l	
Globulins	21–36 g/l	

Table 2.4. (cont.)

	Normal range		Notes
	Male	Female	
IgA	0.5–3.0 g/l		
IgG	5–14 g/l		
IgM	0.5–2.0 g/l		
Creatinine phosphokinase	> 180 IU/l		
Iron	14–32 µmol/l	11–29 µmol/l	
Cholesterol	4.1–9.0 mmol/l (young)		
	5.2–9.0 mmol/l (elderly)		
Triglyceride	0.8–1.7 mmol/l		
Magnesium	0.7–0.95 mmol/l		
Copper	14–22 µmol/l		
Ceruloplasmin	0.3–0.6 g/l		
Immunology			
Rheumatoid factor			
Latex	< 20		
Rose–Waaler	< 32		
Nephelometry	< 40		
ANF	< 1/40		Pattern of immunofluorescence may be helpful (see Chapter 3)
DNA binding	< 30%		
Complement			
C_3	0.55–1.2 g/l		
C_4	0.15–0.5 g/l		
Immune complexes $C1_q$	0–20%		

CSF
Protein 0.15–0.4 g/l
Lymphocytes up to 4/mm³
Glucose 2.5–3.9 mmol/l

Synovial fluid

	Normal	OA	Inflammatory arthritis
Volume (ml)	< 3.5	> 3.5	> 3.5
Viscosity	v. high	high	low
WBC/mm³	< 200	200–2000	2000–100 000
Neutrophils (%)	< 25	< 25	> 50

Urine

Creatinine clearance	> 80 ml/min/m²	Microscopy and urinalysis. The sample should be fresh, centrifuged and a drop of the sediment examined under the microscope. Should be performed daily in active glomerulonephritis
Total protein excretion	< 0.2/24 h	
Na	80–200 mmol/l	
K	30–150 mmol/l	
Hydroxyproline (total)	22–77 mg/24 h	
Calcium	2.5/7.5 mmol/l/24 h	2.5–6.25 mmol/24 h
Phosphate	32–64 mmol/l/24 h	
Homogentisic acid	0	Found in ochronosis

Table 2.4. (cont.)

	Normal range		Notes
	Male	Female	
Haemosiderin	0		If positive indicative of haemolytic anaemia
Schilling test			Malabsorbtion in systemic sclerosis
Stage I	> 12% excretion		
Stage II	> 12% excretion		
Faeces			
24 h fat content	< 5 g/24 h		High in steatorrhoea associated with systemic sclerosis
	18 mmol/24 h		

2 Investigation of rheumatic disease

2.2 Other biochemical and haematological tests

Crystal examination
This is performed using a polarizing light microscope with a first order red compensator. It is important for the clinician to be familiar with the use of the microscope and to have the facility to examine fresh synovial fluids.

Urate crystals are needle shaped and appear yellow parallel to the axis of the red compensator, blue when perpendicular to the axis. They are often numerous, may be seen within white cells and dissolve with uricase.

Calcium pyrophosphate dihydrate crystals are pleomorphic, predominantly rhomboid shaped and have the opposite orientation to urate crystals. They may be scanty and may be found in acute pseudogout and in association with chrondrocalcinosis and osteoarthritis.

Calcium hydroxyapatite crystals may be found in synovial fluids, especially in fluids from patients with osteoarthritis, as well as in periarticular and subcutaneous deposits.
  The crystals are poorly birefringent and are best identified by the use of Alizarin Red staining, which demonstrates them as amorphous clumps of red staining material. Definitive identification may be performed using infra-red spectroscopy and X-ray diffraction.

Cholesterol crystals are very attractive, strongly birefringent crystals and rectangular in shape with one corner cut out. They are soluble in ethanol. They may be found in RA joint fluids especially in the shoulder in patients with chronic disease, as well as in the necrotic centre of the rheumatoid nodule or in the contents of a synovial cyst. Joint fluid containing cholesterol crystals can be difficult to aspirate and may resemble pus.

2 Investigation of rheumatic disease

2.2 Other biochemical and haematological tests

Biochemical studies

Glucose. Synovial fluid glucose should be interpreted with a simultaneous plasma sample. In septic or tuberculous arthritis the synovial fluid glucose will be less than half the serum value. Occasionally low values are seen in RA.

Lactate. Synovial fluid lactate when elevated may be helpful in confirming the presence of infection. However, it is usually normal in gonococcal septic arthritis and treated septic arthritis.

Immunological tests

Tests for rheumatoid factor may be positive in the synovial fluid before the blood.

3 Imaging in the rheumatic diseases

3 Imaging in the rheumatic diseases

Radiography
X-rays should be interpreted in the context of the history and physical examination. A specific diagnosis is seldom possible, but X-rays are useful in the detection and assessment of abnormalities and their changes with time.

Look for soft tissue swelling or for calcification changes in the joint 'space', or thickness of articular cartilage, juxta-articular erosions and other changes such as osteoporosis, fractures, periosteal reactions, subluxation and ankylosis.

Many radiological abnormalities are painless. For example, intervertebral disc space narrowing or the presence of osteophytes in the spine do not necessarily explain a patient's back pain as such changes are common in the middle aged and elderly without complaints.

Specific radiographic appearances in different rheumatic conditions are considered in Chapter 5.

Synoviography
This gives information about the intra-articular anatomy. It is safe, simple and informative. Double contrast techniques are particularly useful in the diagnosis of derangements of the knee and shoulder. Also demonstrated are:
- Acute synovial rupture (ruptured Baker's cyst), helping discriminate this from deep vein thrombosis of the calf, which it resembles clinically. Sometimes a simultaneous venogram will be needed.
- Synovial cysts connecting with joints.
- Connections between joints, bursae and tendon sheaths (especially around the shoulder, wrist and ankle).
- The size of a synovial cavity, the state of its lining, the presence of fibrin deposits, loose bodies or synovial tumours.
- In the knee, tear and displacement of the menisci.
- Lymphatic drainage.

3   Imaging in the rheumatic diseases

Radioisotope scans

Isotopes in the measurement of joint inflammation
Imaging with technetium compounds has been used to detect and quantify inflammation of joints, including the sacroiliac joints, but has not proved reliable.

Recently radioisotope scanning has been found to be predictive of radiographic joint changes in the hands in osteoarthritis and it may prove a helpful adjunct to measurement of disease activity in this condition.

Isotopes in the localization of infection
Gallium-67 citrate is incorporated into neutrophils and localizes at sites of inflammation. It is a good indicator of the presence and location of infection.

Indium-111 labelled neutrophils locate infection in septic arthritis and osteomyelitis.

Miscellaneous uses
Radioisotopes have been used:
- To demonstrate loosening of an articular prosthesis.
- To detect aseptic necrosis of bone before X-ray changes occur.
- To evaluate bone turnover in Paget's disease.
- To demonstrate secondary malignant deposits.
- To diagnose and evaluate osteomalacia.

Computerized axial tomography (CT scans)
CT scans can be used for:
- Assessment of the size of the spinal canal in spinal stenosis.
- Quantative bone densitometry in osteoporosis.
- To provide the earliest evidence of sacroiliitis in ankylosing spondylitis.

Thermography
Thermography measures heat radiation from the skin surface and

3 Imaging in the rheumatic diseases

therefore can be used to measure heat emanating from inflamed joints. Its advantage is that it gives an objective, non-intrusive measurement of inflammation. Applications include:
- Measurement of the response to anti-inflammatory or anti-rheumatic therapy.
- Assessment of the responses to treatment of peripheral Paget's disease.
- Assessment and monitoring of Raynaud's disease.

Bone absorptiometry — dual photon method

This measures bone density and differentiates it from soft tissue density. An isotope source (^{153}Gd) which emits gamma rays of two different energies is placed over the patient and moved in a rectilinear fashion. The softer of the rays is selectively more attenuated by bone. In a modification of this method this isotope is replaced by an X-ray source which uses two different energies. A computer works out the relative densities of bone and soft tissues, compares bone density with population norms and prints a picture.

It is useful in measuring the natural history of post-menopausal and other forms of osteoporosis and the results of treatment.

Advantages over quantative CT include:
- Less expensive.
- Less radiation received.
- It is a dedicated machine and does not have to compete for other uses as with CT scanning.

It is however less sensitive than CT in measuring trabecular bone and misleading information will be given if vertebral compression fractures are present.

Magnetic resonance imaging (MRI)

MRI scanning presents new opportunities for rheumatology by its ability to image soft tissues. The machine is constructed around a large magnet which provides a static magnetic field. A 90°

3 Imaging in the rheumatic diseases

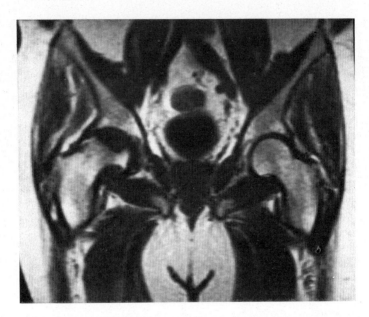

Fig. 3.1 MRI: a T1 weighted transaxial image of the hips showing reduced signal intensity from the superior aspect of the right hip in a patient with osteonecrosis.

pulse is induced by an electromagnetic coil around the patient. The electrical signal resulting from the change in the adjustment of protons in the part to be imaged following the pulse can be detected by a receiver coil and used as a basis for reconstructing the image (Fig. 3.1).

The technique is useful in:
- Upper cervical spine, brain stem and cerebellar pathology, which is poorly imaged by CAT scanning.
- Aseptic necrosis, where it will demonstrate the earliest changes.

3 Imaging in the rheumatic diseases

- In meniscal tears and other internal derangements of the knee.

The potential for providing new information about early joint damage in osteoarthritis and inflammatory conditions is great, but limited by the cost of the machine.

4 Regional problems and soft tissue rheumatism

4.1 Low back pain, 69

4.2 Neck pain, 77

4.3 Shoulder pain, 81

4.4 Soft tissue rheumatism and fibrositis, 85

4.5 Entrapment neuropathies, 91

4 Regional problems and soft tissue rheumatism

4.1 Low back pain

4.1 Low back pain

Low back pain is one of the commonest complaints in patients seen by the rheumatologist or general practitioner. The causes of low back pain are listed in Table 4.1. The history and examination are discussed in Chapter 1.

Table 4.1. Causes of low back pain

1 *No nerve root irritation*
  (a) Vertebral causes:
    Compression fractures — trauma, osteoporosis
    Neoplasia — primary or secondary malignancies
    Infection
    Coccydynia
    Diffuse idiopathic skeletal hyperostosis
    Paget's disease
    Osteoid osteoma
    Congenital defects
      spondylolysis
      spondylolisthesis
      transitional vertebrae
  (b) Intervertebral disc causes:
    Disc herniation and tears of the annulus fibrosis not impinging on the nerves
    Septic discitis, particularly *Staphylococcus aureus* and anaerobic infections
  (c) Apophyseal (facet) joints:
    Lumbar spondylosis
    Rheumatoid arthritis
    Seronegative spondyloarthritis
  (d) Sacroiliitis:
    Ankylosing spondylitis
    Reiter's syndrome
    Psoriatic arthritis
    Ulcerative colitis
    Crohn's disease
    Brucellosis
    Tuberculosis
  (e) Scoliosis
  (f) Referred pain:
    Aortic aneurysm
    Posterior abdominal viscera

4 Regional problems and soft tissue rheumatism

4.1 Low back pain

Table 4.1. (cont.)

    Renal calculi
    Retroperitoneal neoplasms, retroperitoneal fibrosis
 (g) Soft tissues:
    Ligaments and muscles — sprains, tears
    Miscellaneous: fatigue due to poor posture, obesity, neuromuscular disease, inactivity, inequality of leg length

2 *Back pain with nerve root irritation*
 (a) Vertebral causes:
    Spondylolisthesis
    Spondylosis
    Paget's disease
 (b) Intervertebral disc:
    Herniation
 (c) Intra-spinal space-occupying lesions:
    Neurofibroma
    Arachnoid cyst
    Metastatic deposits
    Epidural abscess

3 *Spinal stenosis*

4 *Back pain in children*
 (a) Under 10 years of age:
    Osteoid osteoma
    Fibroma
    Bone cysts
    Ewing's sarcoma
    Osteogenic sarcoma
    Metastases
    Intervertebral disc infection including TB
 (b) Over 10 years of age:
    Spondylolisthesis
    Trauma
    Psychogenic
    Osteochondritis (Scheuermann's disease)
    Juvenile discitis
    Vertebral osteomyelitis

4 Regional problems and soft tissue rheumatism

4.1 Low back pain

Investigations

Caution should be exercised in the interpretation of investigations for low back pain, particularly with the radiographs. Morphological variations become more prevalent with increasing age and the presence of lumbar spondylosis on the radiograph may not necessarily explain the cause of the patient's symptoms.

Laboratory tests
1 Full blood count.
2 Plasma viscosity or ESR.
3 Liver function tests.
4 Serum and urine protein electrophoresis.
5 Calcium and phosphate.

Radiographic examination
1 Plain PA and lateral spinal films.
2 Sacroiliac joints.

Differential diagnosis

In the young adult

Acute back strain presents with diffuse low back pain accompanied by muscle spasm and protective flexion, which are exacerbated by the slightest movement. Examination and investigations are otherwise normal.

Acute disc prolapse often occurs in healthy adults after minimal trauma. Commonly, there is a previous history of back pain or acute strain. The pain is felt initially in the low back and then radiates into the leg associated with paraesthesiae. Exacerbation of pain occurs with coughing or straining. There is severe pain, difficulty with standing, loss of lumbar lordosis, muscular spasm and lumbar scoliosis. Straight leg raising is impaired and

4 Regional problems and soft tissue rheumatism

4.1 Low back pain

neurological signs vary according the nerve roots involved (see Table 1.7). Evidence of bladder or bowel dysfunction suggest cauda equina involvement.

Ankylosing spondylitis presents with lumbar pain associated with stiffness, worse on rest and improved with exercise and NSAIDs. Examination demonstrates loss of lumbar lordosis, restricted back movement and sacroilial pain. X-ray changes may develop later; sacroiliitis, erosion and squaring of the lumbar vertebrae.

Chronic sprain syndrome is common and variable and usually comprises mild backache responsive to rest and exacerbated by lifting and bending. Superimposed episodes of more severe pain radiating into the thighs may occur. Back movements are usually full, although there may be pain at the limits of motion. Loss of motion, muscle spasm, abnormal posture and partial restriction of straight leg raising may occur.

In the late middle aged to elderly

Lumbar spondylosis may resemble the chronic sprain syndrome clinically and is accompanied by radiographic signs of disc degeneration (loss of disc space, evidence of gas within the disc — 'the vacuum sign' — and subchondral sclerosis). Progression may occur to 'degenerative' spondylolisthesis.

'Degenerative' spondylolisthesis has added neurological signs or symptoms secondary to nerve root or cauda equina compression. Radiographs show evidence of lumbar spondylosis with forward displacement of the vertebrae. Oblique views may be required for the detection of milder forms. Figure 4.1 shows spondylolytic spondylolisthesis with a defect in the pars interarticularis.

4 Regional problems and soft tissue rheumatism

4.1 Low back pain

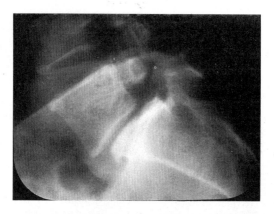

Fig. 4.1 Spondylolisthesis — anterior slipping of L5 on S1 in Grade 1 spondylolytic spondylolisthesis.

Spinal stenosis can be produced by marked spondylolisthesis. The clinical picture is variable; the patient may complain of claudicating type pain in the back and thigh that comes on after walking and is relieved by resting for several minutes. Generalized weakness or numbness and tingling may also occur. Clinical signs may be minimal at rest but demonstrable after walking.

Diffuse idiopathic skeletal hyperostosis (DISH) is ankylosing hyperostosis of the spine affecting the anterolateral aspect of the spine, usually beginning in the thoracic region. Patients may be asymptomatic or complain of mild pain and stiffness in the back as well as other joints. There is a statistical association with diabetes. Radiographs show characteristic large beak-like osteophytes (Fig. 4.2). Fluffy new bone formation may be apparent around the pelvis and calcaneal spurs may occur. Loss of spinal mobility reflects the extent to which the osteophytes of neighbouring vertebrae fuse together, but is rarely total.

4 Regional problems and soft tissue rheumatism

4.1 Low back pain

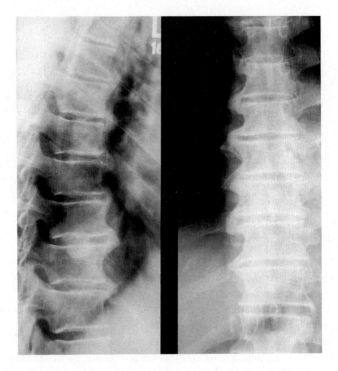

Fig. 4.2 Diffuse idiopathic skeletal hyperostosis showing beak-like osteophytes anterolateral to R vertebral column and relative preservation of disc space height.

Pathological fractures of the vertebral body cause acute back pain that often resolves over a few days. Causes include osteoporosis, metastatic deposits, multiple myeloma and Paget's disease. Bone seeking tumours include lung, breast, thyroid, prostate and adrenal. Pain may be severe and well localized. Plain radiographs should be supplemented by a radioisotope bone scan to look for metastatic deposits, although myeloma requires serum and urine electrophoresis and a bone marrow examination for diagnosis and will not be displayed by the bone scan.

4 Regional problems and soft tissue rheumatism

4.1 Low back pain

All ages

Infection generally presents with severe, localized back pain accompanied by fever. The course of an epidural abscess may be very rapid with progression to paraplegia within 24–48 h. Tuberculous osteomyelitis is characteristically insidious in presentation and the presence of back pain with unexplained weight loss may point to the diagnosis.

Referred pain from abdominal and pelvic viscera. Pain may result from pelvic causes such as retroverted uterus, ovarian disease and salpingitis in women and prostatic lesions in men. Renal stones and pancreatic and other retroperitoneal disease may also cause back pain.

Further investigations
1 Myelography – persistent or increasing neurological problems, herniated disc.
2 Electromyography may confirm neurological involvement.
3 Radioisotope bone scan – infection, metastatic deposits.
4 Computerized axial tomography – spinal stenosis, herniated disc.
5 MRI affords good soft tissue definition in spinal lesions.

Management

Acute strain
Bed rest for 2–3 days. Muscle relaxants, salicylates or NSAIDs may be administered. Narcotic agents may occasionally be required in the acute phase. Heat (moist packs) and light massage help. Some patients respond to manipulative therapy.

Chronic back pain
Bed rest may be helpful in acute exacerbations. Advise about proper sleeping and sitting positions. Physiotherapy and exercise classes improve the strength of back and abdominal muscles.

4 Regional problems and soft tissue rheumatism

4.1 Low back pain

Some pain relief may be obtained from analgesics, shortwave therapy, transcutaneous electrical nerve stimulation and manipulation. Corsets are best avoided as they may lead to wasting of the abdominal and back musculature.

Prolapsed intervertebral disc

Conservative management
Symptoms and signs often resolve with complete bed rest. Other therapeutic modalities may be required and include:
1 Epidural injections (80 mg triamcinalone into the epidural space over 5 min).
2 Traction.
3 Manipulation (in uncomplicated cases).

Surgical management
1 Chemonucleolysis by chymopapain (anaphylaxis may occur in 0.5% of patients).
2 Laminectomy is performed for unresponsive or progressive disease (complications include infective discitis, recurrence of prolapse and spondylolisthesis). Presentation with cauda equina involvement is a medical emergency.
3 Microsurgery techniques for removal of disc prolapse are now available in some centres.

Spondylolisthesis
1 *Minimal symptoms* should be treated by postural exercises.
2 *Severe symptoms* should be treated with spinal fusion, with decompression if neurological signs present.

Spinal stenosis
The patient should be managed conservatively initially. With increasing symptoms surgical decompression is required.

4 Regional problems and soft tissue rheumatism

4.2 Neck pain

4.2 Neck pain

Neck pain is a common source of complaint, but is usually less disabling than back pain (Table 4.2). The history and examination are discussed in Chapter 1.

Investigations

Laboratory tests
1 Full blood count.
2 Plasma viscosity or ESR.
3 Liver function tests.
4 Serum and urine protein electrophoresis.
5 Calcium and phosphate.

Table 4.2. Causes of neck pain

1 *Pain from the cervical spine*
   (a) Osteoarthritis, facet joints usually lower cervical spine
   (b) Rheumatoid arthritis producing atlanto-axial subluxation or vertebral malalignment
   (c) Chronic juvenile arthritis
   (d) Seronegative spondyloarthropathy such as AS and psoriatic arthritis
   (e) Trauma
   (f) Prolapsed intervertebral disc
   (g) Osteomyelitis
   (h) Primary or metastatic tumours
   (i) Epidural abscess

2 *Pain from surrounding structures*
   (a) Acute neck strain
   (b) Torticollis
   (c) Fibrositis
   (d) Sternocleidomastoid tendinitis
   (e) Pharyngeal infection
   (f) Occipital neuritis
   (g) Meningitis and poliomyelitis

4 Regional problems and soft tissue rheumatism

4.2 Neck pain

Radiographic examination
Plain PA and lateral spinal films in flexion and extension. Oblique views may be helpful if neurological features are present.

Differential diagnosis

Acute wry neck occurs unrelated to trauma and severe limitation of movement is accompanied by marked paracervical muscle spasm.

Torticollis. The patient presents with the head held in flexion and rotated to one side by spasm of the sternocleidomastoid muscle.
- A congenital form is painless and associated with swelling of the muscle.
- In young children it is associated with pharyngitis and cervical lymphadenopathy.
- In adults, the condition may be produced by a prolapsed intervertebral disc or following traumatic synovitis of the facet joints. It resolves slowly within 10 days.

Acute neck sprain. There is usually a history of trauma, most commonly a road traffic accident producing a whip-lash injury. Symptoms may be delayed for days to months.

Prolapsed cervical intervertebral disc mainly occurs in young adults following trauma. There may be pain and paraesthesiae radiating to the upper limb (Table 1.6). Direct posterior prolapse is rare and causes features of cord compression.

Meningitis or poliomyelitis is a cause of neck pain in a feverish young child or adult.

Cervical spondylosis accompanied by disc degeneration may

4 Regional problems and soft tissue rheumatism

4.2 Neck pain

give rise to chronic neck pain, often punctuated with episodes of acute neck pain. As each disc degenerates and looses elasticity and height (C5/6 is most often affected) the range of neck movement is reduced and secondary osteophyte formation and strains on the posterior articular facets cause pains which are referred to the appropriate referral areas. These areas differ slightly from the areas of distribution of the corresponding nerve roots.

C4	clavicles
C5	sides of neck to points of shoulders
C6	outer arms
C7	inner arm and axilla

Narrowing of neural foraminae can occur following osteophytic outgrowths from the uncovertebral joints (joints of Luschka) and cause nerve root compression.

Neck pain from any cause activates extensor anti-gravity reflexes with increased tone of sacrospinalis and splenius capitis muscles, associated with 'tension headaches'.

Neck pain due to inflammatory arthropathies. (See appropriate sections.)

Infection, neoplastic involvement of the vertebrae may also be a cause of neck pain.

Further investigations
1 Myelography — persistent or increasing neurological problems with a view to surgery.
2 Electromyography may be used to confirm neurological involvement.
3 Radioisotope bone scan — infection, metastatic deposits.
4 MRI with complex clinical problems as occurs in some patients with severe rheumatoid involvement of the cervical spine.

4 Regional problems and soft tissue rheumatism

4.2 Neck pain

Management

The painful stiff neck (neck strain, wry neck, cervical spondylosis)
Studies indicate that the 1-year recovery rate and outcome are generally favourable and uninfluenced by treatment whether by collar, special pillows, traction, exercises or manipulation. Nevertheless, for the individual, manipulation sometimes brings relief and almost all gain some subjective relief from a collar splint by day and the use of a special neck pillow at night. The latter should be placed in the angle of the neck and shoulder opposite the painful side, on top of the customary pillow. That way it will bring about a gentle stretch of the neck on the most painful side.

NSAIDs in small doses help. Long-term use of a rigid cervical collar leads to neck muscle weakness and is to be avoided.

The stiff neck with neurological involvement
Signs of cord compression (sensory level, limb weakness) constitute a *medical emergency*. Evidence of nerve root involvement should lead to joint management with the orthopaedic surgeons.

4 Regional problems and soft tissue rheumatism

4.3 Shoulder pain

Pain may be referred from the neck, upper ribs or diaphragm (pleurisy, pericarditis, subphrenic abscess). Referred pain is unaffected by movements of the shoulder joint (Table 4.3). The history and examination are discussed in Chapter 1.

Table 4.3. Causes of shoulder pain

1 *Pain from the glenohumeral joint*
   (a) Inflammatory arthropathies such as RA, AS
   (b) Septic arthritis
   (c) Variants of OA associated with pyrophosphate crystals (pyrophosphate arthropathy) and hydroxyapatite crystals (Milwakee shoulder, idiopathic destructive arthritis)
   (d) Aseptic necrosis and barotrauma (Caïsson disease)
   (e) Gout
   (f) Haemophilia
   (g) Neuropathic joint secondary to syringomyelia

2 *Pain from the acromioclavicular joint*
   (a) Inflammatory arthropathies, RA, AS
   (b) OA
   (c) Septic arthritis

3 *Pain from the surrounding soft tissues*
   (a) Adhesive capsulitis (frozen shoulder), shoulder–hand syndrome
   (b) Rotator cuff tears
   (c) Supraspinatus tendinitis
   (d) Calcific periarthritis
   (e) Impingement syndrome
   (f) Bicipital tendinitis
   (g) Subacromial bursitis
   (h) Polymyalgia rheumatica
   (i) Fibrositis

4 *Referred pain*
   (a) Brachial neuritis secondary to cervical spine disease
   (b) Pulmonary embolus
   (c) Cholecystitis
   (d) Subphrenic abscess
   (e) Pancoast tumour

4 Regional problems and soft tissue rheumatism

4.3 Shoulder pain

Differential diagnosis

Rotator cuff tendinitis. Minor trauma on top of a long history of minor shoulder problems may precipitate the pain, often in a man in his 50s. The pain is often poorly localized, may radiate to the mid upper arm, is worse lying on the affected side, and interferes with sleep. Examination reveals a painful arc.

Bicipital tendinitis. Anterior shoulder pain may radiate into the arm. Yergason's test is positive (see section 1.2).

Subacromial bursitis presents in the same way as rotator cuff tendinitis.

Acute calcific tendinitis presents in a patient in the fifth decade with sudden, severe pain in the shoulder often following minor trauma. Movement is restricted and very painful.

Adhesive capsulitis. Gradual onset of pain and limitation of movement. The patient is unable to lie on the affected side and sleep is disturbed. On examination, all movement of the shoulder is restricted and painful.

Shoulder–hand syndrome (algodystrophy, reflex sympathetic dystrophy syndrome). A severe adhesive capsulitis with pain and swelling in the fingers, with vasomotor changes. It may follow myocardial syndrome, subarachnoid haemorrhage, herpes zoster or thoracotomy. Pain is severe and burning. Eventually there may be atrophy of the skin and subcutaneous tissues with contractures. Radiographs show patchy osteoporosis, and there is increased uptake in the affected extremity on bone scan.

Glenohumeral arthritis (RA, AS, osteonecrosis, sepsis). There may be features of an associated rheumatic disease. Pain and restriction of shoulder movement may be accompanied by

4 Regional problems and soft tissue rheumatism

4.3 Shoulder pain

anterior swelling of the shoulder. External rotation is a pure glenohumeral movement and will be limited.

Acromioclavicular arthritis commonly occurs in sportsmen. There is bony enlargement and tenderness of the joint and pain at higher degrees of elevation.

Investigations

Synovial fluid aspiration. Examine for bacteria, cells, crystals.

Radiography will show fractures, dislocations, calcific deposits (calcific periarthritis), may demonstrate glenohumeral pathology (erosions in OA, osteonecrosis), osteoarthritic changes in the acromioclavicular joint, patchy osteoporosis of affected limb in shoulder–hand syndrome, may reveal neck abnormalities in referred pain.

Arthrography will confirm rotator cuff rupture.

Bone scanning demonstrates early osteonecrosis and will show increased uptake in the affected limb in the shoulder–hand syndrome.

Arthroscopy to visualize rotator cuff defects.

Management

Periarthritis syndromes
Rotator cuff tendinitis, bicipital tendinitis, subacromial bursitis are self-limiting and resolve with rest. Recovery may be speeded by local injections of depot corticosteroids and physiotherapy to regain full range of motion. Small doses of analgesics or NSAIDs can be helpful. Rotator cuff or bicipital tendon rupture requires surgical repair in younger, active patients.

4 Regional problems and soft tissue rheumatism

4.3 Shoulder pain

Adhesive capsulitis. Treatment follows the lines outlined above. Hot packs and other forms of heat help relieve pain. Active physiotherapy is best limited to resisted and isometric exercises within the tolerated range. After 6 or 9 months consider manipulation under anaesthetic, which may restore range of movement and relieve pain once it is clear that the condition has become stable. Spontaneous recovery also occurs but may be delayed for 18 months or more.

Shoulder—hand syndrome should be managed as adhesive capsulitis. The prognosis is related to the duration of symptoms and is best influenced by intensive therapy instituted early on. For those not responding within 1 to 4 weeks, sympathetic blockade and/or a short course of steroids (40 mg of oral prednisolone for 2 weeks and tapering over a further 2 weeks) should be considered.

Acute calcific periarthritis is managed as described in section 5.5.

Glenohumeral and acromioclavicular arthritis
This often responds to intra-articular injection of depot corticosteroids once infection has been excluded along with general management of the underlying rheumatic disease. The management of osteonecrosis is described on p. 179—180.

4 Regional problems and soft tissue rheumatism

4.4 Soft tissue rheumatism and fibrositis

4.4 Soft tissue rheumatism and fibrositis

Soft tissue rheumatism is a way of categorizing all those painful rheumatic complaints which do not primarily involve bones and joints.

Fibrositis (fibromyalgia, fibromyositis)

These names implicate inflammation of fibrous tissue or muscles, which on biopsy do not exist. The symptoms, however, are real and consist of increased tenderness felt usually in a stereotyped distribution, which when severe enough is associated with persistent spontaneous pain. Symptoms usually occur against a background of sleep disturbance and mood changes with easy tearfulness. Smythe's group has mapped the main tender points (Fig. 4.3) and tabulated them (Table 4.4).

So-called fibrositis nodules are in reality tender muscle bundles near their insertion into bone. They may be found especially in the:

trapezius;
supraspinatus (along the spine of the scapula);
rhomboids and levator scapulae muscles (along their scapula insertions).

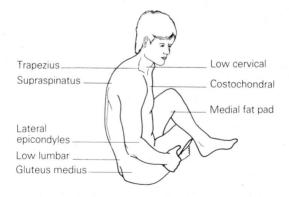

Fig. 4.3 Tender sites found in fibrositis (from Smythe, 1979).

4 Regional problems and soft tissue rheumatism

4.4 Soft tissue rheumatism and fibrositis

Table 4.4. The point count in fibrositis: 14 tender sites (condensed from Smythe, 1979)

Trapezius	Midpoint of upper fold
Costochondral	Maximal on superior aspect, just lateral to 2nd costochondral junction
Lateral epicondyles	1–2 cm distal to lateral epicondyle within the tensed extensor digitorum longus muscle
Supraspinatus	At origins, above scapular spine, near medial border
Low cervical	Anterior aspects of intertransverse spaces C4–7
Low lumbar	Interspinous ligaments L4–S1
Gluteus medius	Upper outer quadrants of buttocks, in anterior fold of muscle
Medial fat pad	Overlying medial collateral ligament of the knee, proximal to joint line

Pain from these areas may radiate into the neck, shoulder and arm. Other tender areas include:
- Origins of sternocleidomastoid and splenius capitis muscles along the superior nuchal line at the occiput. Pain may be felt in the occiput and referred behind the eyes (tension headache).
- Muscle insertions along the lower lumbar and sacral spinous processes, sacral triangle and posterior iliac crests. Pain may be felt in the low back and referred to the buttock, thigh and over the greater trochanter.

Before diagnosing fibrositis:
exclude other pathology causing referred pain and tenderness;
look for a history of sleep disturbance, especially with fatigue on waking;
ask for underlying mood changes with easy tearfulness;
demonstrate the typical tender points.

4 Regional problems and soft tissue rheumatism

4.4 Soft tissue rheumatism and fibrositis

Differential diagnosis
1 Inflammatory conditions:
prodrome of RA or SLE;
polymyalgia rheumatica;
polymyositis.
2 Neoplastic:
multiple myeloma;
bony metastases — secondaries from breast and prostate.
3 Endocrine and metabolic:
hypothyroidism;
osteomalacia.
4 Neurological:
dystonic phase of Parkinson's disease.

Treatment
1 Reassurance, together with a recognition that the symptoms are real.
2 Symptomatic — warming salves and embrocations, local massage and vibromassage.
3 'Trigger spots' may respond to local injection with local anaesthetic–corticosteroid mixtures.
4 A course of low-dose antidepressant may help to reverse sleep disturbances and encourage muscle relaxation.

Tendinitis, enthesitis and bursitis

Flexor tenosynovitis (trigger finger)
One or more of the flexor tendon sheaths of the hand are affected.

The patient will complain of intermittent locking of the finger in flexion requiring manual extension often accompanied by pain.

A nodule is frequently palpable along the course of the tendon sheath in the palm.

Treatment is by infiltration of the tendon sheath with a small

4 Regional problems and soft tissue rheumatism

4.4 Soft tissue rheumatism and fibrositis

amount of corticosteroid (section 7.1). Recurrence is common and may require surgical excision of the stenosed part of the tendon sheath.

de Quervain's tenosynovitis
Involves the tendon sheaths of the abductor pollicis longus and extensor pollicis brevis. Pain is felt in the anatomical snuffbox and Finkelstein's test is positive (see section 1.2). Treatment is as above.

Lateral epicondylitis (tennis elbow)
This is an enthesitis affecting the common insertion of the extensors of the wrist and finger extensors.

Pain is felt in the elbow and may radiate downward into forearm and back of the hand and upwards towards the shoulder.

Tenderness located just distal to the lateral epicondyle. Pain is reproduced on resisted dorsiflexion of the wrist with the elbow at 90°. (See Cozen's test p. 22)

Treatment is by local injection of a corticosteroid/lignocaine mixture (section 7.1). The patient should be warned that the pain may increase for 24 h or so before improving. The arm should be rested. Ultrasound may prove successful in some cases; splints and surgical procedures are used when other treatments have failed.

Medial epicondylitis (golfer's elbow)
This is caused by enthesitis affecting the common tendon insertion of the flexors of the hand and wrist.

Pain is felt around the medial aspect of the elbow. Tenderness is localized to the region of epicondyle and reproduced by resisted wrist flexion.

Treatment is as for tennis elbow but beware the nearby ulnar nerve.

4 Regional problems and soft tissue rheumatism

4.4 Soft tissue rheumatism and fibrositis

Subacromial bursitis (see section 4.3)

Trochanteric bursitis. This involves the bursae around the gluteal insertion at the greater trochanter of the femur.

Pain is felt on the lateral hip and thigh and is often exacerbated by lying on the affected side.

Tenderness is localized to the greater trochanter and is increased by resisted abduction of the hip.

Treatment is with wide infiltration of corticosteroids and lignocaine.

Ischial bursitis. Inflammation of the bursa between the gluteus maximus and the ischial tuberosity causing pain localized to the area.

Treatment as above, but avoid the sciatic nerve, which passes midway between the ischial tuberosity and the greater trochanter.

Other forms of bursitis

Anserine bursitis. This involves the sartorius bursa on the medial upper tibia. It may cause pain especially when climbing stairs.

Olecranon bursitis. A fluctuant swelling, often painless over the olecranon. It is inflamed as a consequence of trauma, pressure, gout, infection or rheumatoid arthritis. In rheumatoid arthritis, nodules occur in the bursa wall and in gout, tophi are seen.

Pre-patella bursitis (housemaid's knee). This is often a traumatic lesion, but is also seen in rheumatoid arthritis and other causes in inflammatory arthritis. Infection should be excluded before injection of corticosteroids.

4   Regional problems and soft tissue rheumatism

4.4   Soft tissue rheumatism and fibrositis

Achilles bursitis is often seen in HLA B27-related conditions and rheumatoid arthritis. It leads to erosion of the underlying calcaneum. As in treatment of achilles tendinitis other forms of treatment are tried first (rest, ultrasound, non-steroidal anti-inflammatory drugs, radiotherapy) before local corticosteroid injection, as tendon rupture is a feared complication.

Calcaneal bursitis affects the bursa related to the insertion of the plantar fascia to the os calcis. It may respond to local corticosteroids, but the injection is frequently very painful.

Repetitive strain injury (RSI)
This is a syndrome of occupational importance characterized by:
1 Complaint of pain building up in the forearm on continued use of the fingers, sometimes considered to be a form of tendinitis.
2 Occurrence mainly in young women employed in the communication industries, operating computer and other keyboards.
3 Expressions of feelings of resentment and hostility. There is usually a compensation element.

It has only rarely been reported in other occupations requiring repetitive finger movement such as professional violin or piano playing.

4 Regional problems and soft tissue rheumatism

4.5 Entrapment neuropathies

4.5 Entrapment neuropathies

Carpal tunnel syndrome
Compression of the median nerve at the wrist is the commonest of the entrapment neuropathies.

Aetiology
1 Idiopathic (most common).
2 Inflammatory conditions:
   inflammatory arthopathies such as rheumatoid arthritis;
   sepsis.
3 Endocrine changes:
   pregnancy;
   hypothyroidism;
   acromegaly.
4 Traumatic, following fracture.
5 Infiltrative disorders;
   amyloidosis.

Clinical features
Pain, tingling and thermal paraesthesia in the hand in the distribution of the median nerve. Sometimes the paraesthesia component is absent and may cause diagnostic difficulty especially in a patient with rheumatoid arthritis. Pain frequently radiates into the forearm.

Nocturnal exacerbation is common; the patient may hang an arm out of the bed to relieve the symptoms.

Later numbness may develop in the palm and palmar surface of lateral 3½ digits followed by weakness and wasting of the muscles of the thenar eminence.

Tinel's and Phalen's tests are often positive (see section 1.2).

Diagnostic tests
Therapeutic relief may be produced by the injection of a small amount of corticosteroid into the carpal tunnel (see section 7.1).

4 Regional problems and soft tissue rheumatism

4.5 Entrapment neuropathies

Electrodiagnosis may be helpful in difficult cases where corticosteroids have failed or are not indicated.

Treatment
1 Local injection of corticosteroid.
2 Wrist splint.
3 Surgical decompression.

Other entrapment neuropathies

The ulnar nerve. Entrapment occurs as it passes behind the medial epicondyle of the elbow, through a fascial tunnel. This is more likely to occur where there has been joint swelling or previous injury (tardive ulnar palsy).

Clinical features: radial deviation of the hand, wasting of the hypothenar eminence with blunting of sensation in the medial 1½ digits.

Treatment: surgical re-routing of the ulnar nerve.

Cervical rib and thoracic outlet syndrome. Compression of the lower roots of the brachial plexus may occur as they arch over the thoracic outlet. Cervical ribs or fascial bands may be the cause, but symptoms may occur in their absence.

Clinical features: pain in the arm and weakness of the hands, particularly in the small muscles supplied by T1 and occasionally some weakness of the forearm flexors and extensors.

Diagnosis and treatment: nerve conduction studies. Treatment is surgical.

In the vascular form of the thoracic outlet syndrome, the brachial artery is compressed in certain positions of the shoulder. A characteristic presenting symptom is claudication-like pain in the arm in a woman carrying a heavy shopping basket. The Adson test may be helpful in diagnosis (see section 1.2).

Meralgia paraesthetica is caused by the compression of the

4 Regional problems and soft tissue rheumatism

4.5 Entrapment neuropathies

lateral cutaneous nerve of the thigh as it passes through the lateral part of the inguinal ligament. It is more common in obese or pregnant women.

Clinical features: presents as a patch of painful paraesthesia along the antero-lateral thigh.

Treatment: injection of local corticosteroid around the nerve at the inguinal ligament. Surgical decompression may be required but is not invariably successful.

The lateral popliteal nerve may be compressed as it winds round the neck of the fibula.

Clinical features: sensory changes of antero-lateral aspect of the leg and foot, extending medially to the junction between the fourth and fifth toes. Weakness may occur in the dorsiflexor muscles of the toes and foot and the peroneal muscles leading to foot drop with inversion.

Treatment: surgical decompression.

Tarsal tunnel syndrome is analogous to the carpal tunnel syndrome occurring at the wrist caused by compression of posterior tibial nerve.

Clinical features: pain may be felt in the foot and may be reproduced by percussion of the nerve at the medial malleolus.

Treatment: corticosteroid injection into the tarsal tunnel or surgical decompression.

Morton's metatarsalgia is thought to be due to compression of the plantar digital nerve between the metatarsal heads, most commonly being seen between the second and third digits. A neuroma may form.

Clinical features: pain in the foot on walking with local tenderness at the site of compression. Sensory loss in one or both toes may occur.

Treatment: surgical excision.

5 Important rheumatological conditions

5.1 Rheumatoid arthritis, 97

5.2 Osteoarthritis, 113

5.3 Seronegative spondylarthropathies, 122

5.4 Connective tissue diseases, 137

5.5 The crystal arthropathies, 150

5.6 Polymyalgia rheumatica and giant cell arteritis, 165

5.7 Bone disease, 170

5.8 Infective arthritis, 186

5.9 Trauma and haemorrhage, 198

5.10 Paediatric rheumatology, 201

5.11 The vasculitides, 207

5.12 Rarer rheumatic syndromes, 218

5 Important rheumatological conditions

5.1 Rheumatoid arthritis

5.1 Rheumatoid arthritis

RA is a systemic disease most commonly presenting as a symmetrical polyarthritis. It is the most common of the inflammatory arthropathies and occurs in 2% of the adult population. Eighty per cent of patients have a positive test for rheumatoid factor. Peak ages of onset are between 35 and 45 years but any age can be affected.

Pathogenesis
- Genetic — 70% of patients with RA are HLA DR4 positive.
- Immunological processes. Immune complexes form in the joint which activate and fix complement and attract neutrophils. The neutrophils ingest the immune complexes triggering the release of prostaglandins and other mediators of inflammation.
- The synovium proliferates, hypertrophies and forms granulation tissue (pannus).
- Pannus erodes cartilage and bone.
- Extra-articular manifestations may represent deposition of systemic immune complexes.

Pathology
The changes in the synovial membrane are:
- Hyperplasia and multiplication of the surface cells.
- Infiltration of the subsynovial layers with lymphocytes and plasma cells.
- The synovial tissue becomes thickened and develops a villous appearance with increased vascularity. The changes are not specific for RA.
- The thickened synovium or pannus grows across cartilage and invades bone ends to produce erosions.

Tendon sheath and bursal linings show similar chronic inflammatory changes and tendons may be subject to nodule formation, adhesion, rupture and dislocation. Bursitis may also develop.

5 Important rheumatological conditions

5.1 Rheumatoid arthritis

Clinical features

Onset of symptoms is typically insidious, comprising systemic features such as malaise and weight loss as well as joint pain and swelling, with early morning stiffness.

Other modes of onset include:
- Acute synovitis, onset may be overnight.
- Polymyalgic, presenting mainly as muscular aching and stiffness (especially the elderly).
- Palindromic, recurrent episodes of synovitis returning to normal in between.
- Monoarthritis, occasionally presenting as a monarticular arthritis of the knee.

Joints

RA becomes a symmetrical polyarthritis mainly affecting the small joints of the hands (MCPs and PIPs with sparing of the DIPs), the wrists, knees, feet, ankles, shoulders and elbows.

Hands and wrists. (Wrists 85%, MCP joints 80%, PIP joints 60%). Initial features are of pain and swelling of the MCP and PIP joints with inability to make a fist. Later, involvement at the wrist produces volar subluxation of the hand with radial deviation giving rise to compensatory ulnar deviation of the fingers. Dorsal subluxation of the distal ulnar may be complicated by tendon rupture either by synovial involvement of the tendon or by erosion against bony spicules that form in the distal ulnar head. Inflammation within the carpal tunnel may give rise to carpal tunnel syndrome. Other features include:

MCP joints	swelling, capsular laxity, subluxation
PIP joints	swelling (spindling), hyperextension (swan neck deformity),
	fixed flexion deformity (Boutonnière deformity)
tendons	tenosynovitis, adhesions, nodules, trigger finger

5 Important rheumatological conditions

5.1 Rheumatoid arthritis

Feet and ankles (feet 80%, ankles 70%). MTP joint synovitis may be apparent by the presence of 'daylight' between the toes and tenderness to MTP 'squeezing'. Later, subluxation may occur, causing the patient to feel as though she is walking on pebbles. Involvement of the subtaloid joint at the ankle causes valgus deformity of the forefoot.

Knees (80%). Synovitis, prepatellar bursitis, effusions, Baker's cyst, synovial rupture, valgus or varus deformities, instability and quadriceps wasting are all features.

Elbows (70%). Loss of full extension is a common sign in rheumatoid arthritis.

Shoulders (60%). Subacromial bursitis and rotator cuff lesions commonly occur as well as glenohumeral joint involvement.

Cervical spine (35%). Synovitis of the uncovertebral joints, atlanto-axial subluxation, subaxial subluxation.

Hips (27%). Less often involved, but in severe cases (about 5%) leading to erosion with remodelling of the acetabulum (protrusio acetabuli).

Others include temporomandibular joints (20%), sternoclavicular and manubriosternal joints although almost any synovial joints may become involved including the cricoarytenoids.

Extra-articular manifestations
1 Malaise, lethargy, depression, weight loss.
2 Rheumatoid nodules — subcutaneous nodules over the extensor surfaces of the forearm, sacrum, heel pad, tendon sheaths.
3 Bone — osteoporosis.
4 Eyes — keratoconjunctivitis sicca, scleritis, keratolysis, scleromalacia, scleromalacia perforans.

5 Important rheumatological conditions

5.1 Rheumatoid arthritis

5 Cardiovascular system — pericarditis, pericardial effusions, constrictive pericarditis, tamponade, myocarditis, nodules (pericardial, valves, conduction pathways).
6 Respiratory system — pleural effusions, pleurisy, nodules (subpleural or intraparenchymal), Caplan's syndrome (coal worker's pneumoconiosis with rheumatoid nodules in the lung), fibrosing alveolitis, pulmonary hypertension, obliterative bronchiolitis.
7 Nervous system — entrapment neuropathies (most often median nerve), peripheral neuropathy, mononeuritis multiplex (in vasculitis), cervical cord compression, nerve root compression.
8 Haematological — anaemia, thrombocytopenia, lymphadenopathy (early disease), Felty's syndrome (neutropenia and splenomegaly).
9 Vasculitis — small, medium vessels, digital infarcts, gangrene, mononeuritis multiplex (see section 5.11), leg ulcers.
10 Sjögrens syndrome — dry eyes and mouth (see Chapter 5.4).

In the majority of patients, arthritis is the most prominent feature, but many have extra-articular manifestations. These manifestations are associated with positive tests for rheumatoid factor and may not correlate with the presence or activity of arthritis.

Investigations

Laboratory tests (see also Chapter 2)
1 Raised ESR — often greater than 100 mm/h and correlates with the size and number of affected joints and activity of disease.
2 Elevated plasma viscosity.
3 Raised CRP.
4 Anaemia is common:
  normo/hypochromic normocytic anaemia of chronic disease;

5 Important rheumatological conditions

5.1 Rheumatoid arthritis

hypochromic, microcytic with iron deficiency (e.g. due to GI bleeding);

thrombocytosis is common in active disease;

neutropenia found with drug therapy or in Felty's syndrome.

5 Rheumatoid factor is positive in 80%; positives occur in 30% of related disease such as SLE, DM, SS and PAN.

6 Antinuclear factor positive in 20%.

7 Synovial fluid is inflammatory with 2000–50 000 cells/mm^3.

X-rays (most helpful for diagnosis)

Hands and feet. Aid diagnosis, prognosis and disease monitoring. Earliest erosions may be seen on the foot radiograph.

X-ray changes include:

soft tissue swelling;

juxta-articular osteoporosis;

marginal erosions;

deformities.

With more chronic disease, soft tissue swelling and juxta-articular osteoporosis may be less prominent (Fig. 5.1).

Cervical spine. Required for neck symptoms and prior to neck surgery. Flexion and extension films are helpful and may show:

subluxation of the atlanto-axial joint:

anterior, due to laxity of the transverse ligament;

posterior, with fracture or destruction of the odontoid peg (Fig. 5.2);

upward;

stepladdering of the cervical spine (Fig. 5.2).

Tomography may help with visualization of the odontoid peg.

Chest X-ray for cardiac and respiratory complications of RA (Fig. 5.3).

5 Important rheumatological conditions

5.1 Rheumatoid arthritis

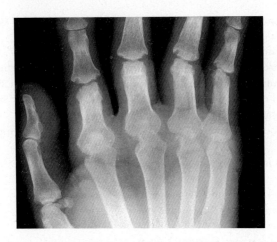

Fig. 5.1 Old rheumatoid disease showing well-defined erosions, absence of osteoporosis and swelling, and foreshortening of proximal phalanges due to Boutonniere deformity.

CT scanning and MRI
Helpful in the preoperative evaluation of a patient with complicated neck disease.

Biopsy
Biopsy of a nodule (central necrosis surrounded by a characteristic palisading cellular area) or synovium (lymphocytes, plasma cells with occasional giant cells infiltrating enlarged villi) may also be helpful in difficult cases.

Differential diagnosis

Rheumatoid arthritis usually presents as an evolving disease, and often requires a period of observation until the whole picture emerges. For this reason, many of the inflammatory arthropathies may mimic rheumatoid arthritis especially in its early stages. However, some conditions can be mistaken for rheumatoid arthritis for some years.

5 Important rheumatological conditions

5.1 Rheumatoid arthritis

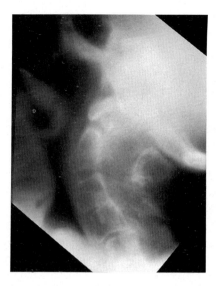

Fig. 5.2 Rheumatoid neck disease. Tomogram shows eroded fragmented odontoid peg, backward displacement of C1 arch on neck extension, and minor stepladdering of C4 on C5.

Osteoarthritis. Elderly patients with the pyrophosphate variant of OA may show 'pseudo-rheumatoid' appearances of the hand with wrist involvement together with prominence of the 2nd and 3rd MCP joint. Distinguish by lack of synovial thickening, reversible 'deformities', radiological appearances and lack of rheumatoid factor.

Psoriatic arthritis. One presentation of psoriatic arthropathy resembles RA clinically. Note skin rash, nail and DIP joint involvement, proliferative erosions on the radiograph and absence of rheumatoid factor and subcutaneous nodules.

Gout. Chronic tophaceous gout occasionally resembles RA clinically. Diagnosis relies on demonstration of hyperuricaemia

5 Important rheumatological conditions

5.1 Rheumatoid arthritis

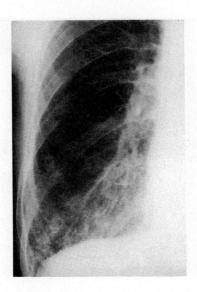

Fig. 5.3 Rheumatoid lung: honeycomb lung in advanced pulmonary fibrosis associated with rheumatoid arthritis.

with uric acid crystals from tophi. Radiographs may also be helpful.

Systemic lupus erythematosus. Prominent systemic component (i.e. visceral organs and CNS), serositis, photosensitive rash with mild non-erosive synovitis. Serology demonstrates high titre ANA and anti-dsDNA antibodies.

Complications
1 Amyloidosis. Suspect this in RA patients who develop proteinuria. Rectal biopsy should be performed.
2 Septic arthritis. RA patients, particularly those with long-standing disease on corticosteroids have an increased risk of

5 Important rheumatological conditions

5.1 Rheumatoid arthritis

infection of their joints. Suspect this whenever an unexpected acute monarthritis or an asymmetrical flare occurs. Confirm the diagnosis by synovial and blood cultures.

Management
Only principles of management are discussed here. For further information see Chapter 6. No curative therapy is available, but much can be done. The following aims or goals should be established.
- Correct diagnosis and assessment of the severity of disease.
- Education of patient and caring relatives.
- Induction of remission by using analgesic/anti-inflammatory and disease modifying drugs.
- Maintenance of joint function, muscle strength and prevention of deformities.
- Correction of joint damage to relieve pain, improve function or correct contractures.

For the hospital patient, successful management involves a team approach: this includes the rheumatologist, general practitioner, surgeon, occupational therapist, physiotherapist, social worker, nurse and family.

Rest
Bed rest in hospital is beneficial for acute arthritis or acute exacerbations of chronic RA. Complete bed rest is reserved for those with early disease, shown by severe inflammatory arthritis and systemic symptoms.

Gradual mobilization and gentle physiotherapy should commence as the patient improves (usually within 1 week).

The aim of splints is to provide rest for inflamed joints. Resting splints support acutely swollen joints in a position of function. Work splints aim to improve function of damaged joints; these are helpful at the wrist.

5 Important rheumatological conditions

5.1 Rheumatoid arthritis

Drug therapy

Analgesic/non-steroidal anti-inflammatory drugs (NSAIDs). These are first line agents used with the aim of reducing pain and inflammation. Many preparations are available and patients respond to different agents in an individual way. For a detailed discussion see section 6.1.

Disease modifying and long-acting drugs. These agents are used when there is persistently active disease despite optimal anti-inflammatory therapy. They should not be used when mechanical problems rather than inflammatory features are a cause of pain or disability. Only three agents have been shown to heal erosions: these include gold, high dose steroid (prednisolone ≥ 12.5 mg), which is no longer used due to unacceptable toxicity and cyclosphophamide, a toxic drug of last resort.

When to use second-line agents?
1 Severe synovitis not responding to NSAIDs alone.
2 The development of erosions on the radiograph (hands or feet).
3 The presence of extra-articular manifestations such as nodules, alveolitis, Felty's syndrome, etc.
4 Not until 1 year of observation (or in very severe disease — 6 months) has revealed no tendency to natural remission.

Which drug should be used? (see Table 5.1)
Practitioners vary in their preferences of disease modifying drugs. Penicillamine and gold are common first choices with sulphasalazine and hydroxychloroquine as alternatives. Resistant patients may then require the use of immunosuppressive agents. Azathioprine and methotrexate are efficacious without being too toxic; cyclophosphamide and chlorambucil are drugs reserved for severe disease and those with life-threatening complications such as systemic vasculitis. Steroids are now mainly used as intra-articular preparations.

5 Important rheumatological conditions

5.1 Rheumatoid arthritis

The order that drugs are chosen depends on the individual patient: a patient with troublesome synovitis may respond to a second line drug with little toxicity such as sulphasalazine, whereas a patient with rapidly deforming, destructive disease may be treated initially with gold or penicillamine, before moving on to methotrexate if there is little response.

How long to treat?
Most patients relapse after stopping disease modifying agents such as penicillamine. It is probably best to continue the drug indefinitely at minimum effective dose, whilst the patient still tolerates it. Unfortunately, efficacy/toxicity is such that very few patients are still taking the same drug 5 years after its initiation.

As the number of disease modifying agents is limited it is important that a fair trial of the agent is given at the reasonable

Table 5.1. Approach to drug management in rheumatoid arthritis

First line
Non-steroidal anti-inflammatory agents
Analgesics

Second line
Hydroxychloroquine
Sulphasalazine
Gold
Penicillamine

Third line
Azathioprine
Methotrexate
Cyclophosphamide
Chlorambucil

Steroids
Intra-articular — useful at any stage
Oral — low dose (5–10 mg) may be used on their own or in combination with disease modifying agents
Parenteral — used to cover surgery or in life-threatening events such as systemic vasculitis (methyl prednisolone)

5 Important rheumatological conditions

5.1 Rheumatoid arthritis

dosage. Inform patients that gold and penicillamine can take up to 3 months before having an effect. Avoid pitfalls such as taking penicillamine with iron medication (which will reduce the absorption of the former). Toxicity does not necessarily entail discontinuation of the drug; it may be enough to reduce dosage. All drugs are discussed fully in section 7.1.

Physical and occupational therapies
These include active exercises, hydrotherapy, application of heat, joint protection classes and assessment of activities of daily living with provision of aids and adaptations (see section 6.2).

Chiropody and foot problems
See section 6.4.

Education and counselling
Common problems are: loss of independence and self-esteem; relations with friends and family can be altered; employment can be threatened. Doctors need to be attentive to the psychological needs of their patients and should help the sufferer to attain a routine and philosophy which makes the burden of disease tolerable.

Surgery
Surgery can reduce pain of a mechanical nature, restore loss of function or correct instability or loss of mobility. Synovectomy halts progression of disease only temporarily. Large joint replacement can give more functional improvement than finger joint surgery. Knee and hip replacements give excellent pain relief. However, the failure rate with the knee is higher than that of the hip. Surgery can be effective in the hand and wrist, but should be performed when the outcome would improve function or quality of life, not just for cosmesis. See also section 6.3.

5 Important rheumatological conditions

5.1 Rheumatoid arthritis

Local injection of corticosteroids (see section 7.1)
These can be a useful adjunct to suppressing a flare of pain and inflammation in a single joint. Injection should be seen as a means whereby the joint can be used actively and the patient take part in physiotherapeutic threatments aimed at maintaining limb strength and mobility. The widespread use of local injection therapy has cut down hospital inpatient time and made most rest splints unnecessary.

Prognosis
The following presenting features indicate a poor prognosis.
- High titre rheumatoid factor at first presentation or within 1 year of onset.
- Early appearance of erosions (within 1 year of onset of symptoms).
- Other extra-articular manifestations.
- HLA DR4.

In the majority of hospital patients adequate control of the disease can be obtained. Only a minority (about one in ten) proceed to severe disability.

Special problems in RA patients

Anaemia
Anaemia of chronic disease (haemoglobin level as low as 8–10 mg/dl) is not uncommon in RA, and usually reflects disease activity. The blood film normally shows a normo/hypochromic, normocytic picture and the serum ferritin is raised reflecting its role as an acute phase reactant.

Iron deficiency anaemia may also occur, often secondary to upper GI bleeding related to therapy with non-steroidal anti-inflammatory agents. Other causes include poor nutrition (especially in the elderly) and GI malignancy.

Pernicious anaemia is another autoimmune disease that occurs

5 Important rheumatological conditions

5.1 Rheumatoid arthritis

more frequently in RA patients. The blood film shows a macrocytic anaemia and blood B_{12} levels are low. The presence of anti-parietal cell antibodies and an abnormal Schilling test help to confirm the diagnosis.

A macrocytic anaemia can also be caused by poor folate intake especially if the patient is also taking methotrexate or sulphasalazine which interfere with folate metabolism. Simple macrocytosis is seen with azathioprine.

Investigations include the following:

a bone marrow examination often helps diagnosis in difficult cases;

upper GI endoscopy if there is an iron deficiency picture present;

lower GI studies may be needed to exclude a neoplasm.

Management of anaemia of chronic disease requires treatment of the underlying condition. There is some evidence that iron therapy may actually increase inflammation in this case. Iron deficiency anaemia may persist with no cause being found despite investigation. Iron supplementation should be given. If the anaemia becomes severe a blood transfusion may be required. If recurrent blood transfusions are needed, then it may be worthwhile investigating for rare causes of bleeding such as angiocaecal dyplasia. However, such patients are often old and the benefits and risks have to be seriously considered.

Vasculitis
See section 5.11.

Leg ulcers
Aetiology may be vasculitic, secondary to stasis and corticosteroid therapy leading to skin atrophy. Pyoderma gangrenosum may also occur.
Management includes the following:
1 Control of underlying cause and treatment of superimposed infection.

5 Important rheumatological conditions

5.1 Rheumatoid arthritis

2 Rest and elevation of the limb.
3 Topical debridement — Debrisan, Sherisorb, Iodosorb (Eusol may damage granulation tissue).
4 Occlusive dressings — Granuflex, Sorbsan (may need frequent changing for profuse exudate).
5 Impregnated dressings — Jelonet, Bactigras — during later stages of healing.
6 Resistant ulcers may require grafting.

Cervical spine involvement
Clinical features include:
1 Symptoms range from neck pain with radiation into the occiput and frontal region to symptoms of cord compression. Be wary of the patient with chronic disease who complains of increasing weakness in the limbs. Drop attacks, incontinence, vertigo and peripheral paraesthesias may also occur.
2 Examine for long tract signs. Upward subluxation causes the odontoid peg to enter the foramen magnum. Loss of corneal reflexes is an early sign (the sensory tract of V descends into the upper cervical region). Nystagmus and pyramidal lesions occur in severe instances.

Treatment consists of:
1 Uncomplicated disease should be managed conservatively with analgesics, non-steroidal anti-inflammatory drugs, neck pillow and cervical collar.
2 Severe pain or neurological involvement requires surgical advice.

Felty's syndrome
This is the association of RA with splenomegaly and neutropenia occurring in about 1% of RA patients.
There is a high frequency of exta-articular features (p. 100).
Common problems include:
recurrent infections, which may be life-threatening; vasculitis; chronic leg ulcers.

5 Important rheumatological conditions

5.1 Rheumatoid arthritis

The cause of the neutropenia is unknown and probably multifactorial. Both humoral and cellular factors have been implicated as well as splenic sequestration of white cells.

Treatment consists of the following.

1 Disease modifying agents are generally indicated. Some investigators have found parenteral gold to be particularly beneficial.

2 Splenectomy is worth considering. The white cell count usually rises to normal after splenectomy. Infections usually respond with considerable improvement in general health; however in some patients there is no improvement.

Pulmonary fibrosis
This disease begins in the lung bases and occurs in 5−10% of RA patients. It may be monitored by symptoms and by CXR, and pulmonary function tests including transfer factor. Disease modifying agents are indicated. Some centres advocate more aggressive regimes with cytotoxic therapy.

5.2 Osteoarthritis

This condition is also known as osteoarthrosis or degenerative joint disease, but as inflammation is often present in the affected joints, for some osteoarthritis (OA) is the preferred terminology.

The hallmark of OA is loss of hyaline cartilage with an accompanying subchondral bone reaction. This leads to the pathological appearances of fibrillation of cartilage, with chondrocyte proliferation and cluster formation. There is increased blood flow in subchondral bone, increased intra-osseous pressure with bone sclerosis, cyst formation and marginal osteophytes.

Aetiology

Two major groups are recognized:

1 Primary OA — no underlying cause found.
2 Secondary OA — associated with various other conditions (see Table 5.2).

It has become clear that even primary OA represents a heterogeneous group of disorders. Epidemiological studies have identified a number of factors which increase the chance of OA occurring.

Age	prevalence increases with age after 50
Sex	under 50 years M > F, the converse is true after 50.
Race	OA hip less common in Asian and Chinese communities
	generalized nodal OA (GOA) rare in Africans
Genetics	autosomal dominant inheritance in GOA
	familial cases of premature OA described
Metabolic	OA associated with obesity, hypertension, hyperuricaemia, hyperlipidaemia and diabetes

Pathogenesis

Advances in joint biochemistry are altering our understanding of the disease so that concepts of a passive 'wear and tear' process are outmoded.

5 Important rheumatological conditions

5.2 Osteoarthritis

Normal cartilage is made up of chondrocytes in an avascular hydrated matrix comprising negatively charged proteoglycan aggregates constrained by a collagen net.

Matrix components are synthesized by the chondrocytes and in OA some as yet unidentified processes alter the balances between synthesis and degradation leading to cartilage loss. The subchondral bone is extremely active, but the relationship between this and the cartilage changes are not known.

Synovial changes are variable and in some forms of crystal-related OA may be marked.

Prevalence
Approximately 5 million people are affected in the UK. OA accounts for seven times as much disability as rheumatoid arthritis.

Clinical features
Several clinical subsets of OA may be recognized.

Generalized nodal OA (GOA)
- Onset in middle-aged Caucasian women, often around the menopause.
- There is a positive family history and a rapid, often inflammatory onset.
- Joints affected include:
  distal interphalangeal (Heberden's nodes);
  proximal interphalangeal (Bouchard's nodes);
  thumb base (1st carpometacarpal);
  spinal apophyseal joints;
  knees;
  1st metatarsophalangeal.

OA of the hip
- More common in men.
- May be due to underlying disorder such as Perthe's disease,

5 Important rheumatological conditions

5.2 Osteoarthritis

acetabular dysplasia, etc.
- Superolateral disease most common, often unilateral, poor prognosis.
- Medial or concentric form associated with polyarticular disease and has a better prognosis.

OA of the knee
- With varus deformity, more common in obese women and certain races e.g. Egyptian, Saudi Arabian. In men it often follows trauma to, or operation on the menisci.

OA associated with crystal deposition
- Calcium pyrophosphate dihydrate crystals.
- Calcium hydroxyapatite (see section 5.5).

Rare disorders
- *Kashin–Beck disease*. Endemic in Eastern Siberia. Severe, polyarticular OA from childhood, associated with fungal infection of grain (*Fusaria sporotrichiella*).
- *Epiphyseal dysplasias*. Familial leading to premature OA. There are various types:
  spondyloepiphyseal dysplasia in which OA of the hip is common:
  multiple epiphyseal dysplasia which exhibits short stature and multiple joint abnormalities.
- *Ochronosis*. Autosomal recessive deficiency of homogentisic acid oxidase. Associated with intervertebral disc calcification (see Fig. 5.4) and premature OA.
Pigmentation of ear cartilage, sclerae, cornea and conjuctivae occurs. The urine turns black on standing or with added alkali. Prolapsed intervertebral disc in 20% of men. Renal and prostatic calcification occur.
- *Haemochromatosis*. Iron storage disorder involving multiple systems. Presentation aged 40–60 years. Diabetes, cirrhosis, skin pigmentation, hypopituitarism may occur.

5 Important rheumatological conditions

5.2 Osteoarthritis

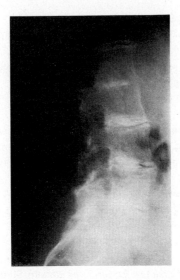

Fig. 5.4 Ochronosis showing extensive disc calcification, gross disc degeneration, and osteopenia throughout the spine.

Arthropathy initially involves 2nd and 3rd MCP joints; may progress to involve wrists, shoulders, elbows, hips, knees, ankles and spine. Pseudogout attacks occur in 50% of patients. Radiographs show prominent involvement of 2nd and 3rd MCP joints, with marked subchondral cysts and other OA changes. Chondrocalcinosis in 50% of patients. Serum ferritin is grossly raised and liver biopsy is diagnostic.

Symptoms and signs in OA
Symptoms include:
    pain on weight bearing and joint movement;
    relieved by rest;
    stiffness is of short duration and confined to involved joints.

5 Important rheumatological conditions

5.2 Osteoarthritis

Signs include:
- bony enlargement;
- localized tenderness;
- crepitus;
- small effusions may be present;
- pain and restriction of movement;
- transient swelling of periarticular structures may occur with inflammatory exacerbations.

Investigations

Blood tests
There are no diagnostic tests. Laboratory tests are performed if the clinical picture is unusual (e.g. premature OA) to exclude a metabolic cause such as haemochromatosis or to exclude other forms of rheumatic disease. These tests include:
- blood count and viscosity (usually normal);
- urea, electrolytes, liver function, calcium and phosphate;
- rheumatoid factor;
- uric acid.

X-rays
Affected joints demonstrate:
- joint space narrowing;
- subchondral sclerosis;
- osteophytosis;
- bony cysts;
- ossicles;
- ankylosis rare.

So-called erosive OA seen in the DIP and PIP joints gives rise to subchondral erosions and a 'gull-wing' appearance on the radiograph (Fig. 5.5).

It is important to note that much radiographic OA is painless and the finding of OA on the radiograph does not prove that the pain is arising in the joint.

5 Important rheumatological conditions

5.2 Osteoarthritis

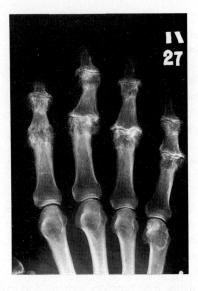

Fig. 5.5 Osteoarthritis of the hands showing involvement of the PIP and DIP joints; joint space narrowing, osteophytosis, subchondral sclerosis and cysts; subchondral erosions seen in 'erosive OA' (and ankylosis in some joints as may occur occasionally).

Management
Many patients with OA can be successfully managed with rest and reassurance. Specific therapy to halt the underlying disease process is not available, but much can be done to reduce symptoms and maximize mobility and independence. A multidisciplinary approach is essential.

Education
Booklets produced by the Arthritis and Rheumatism Council explain the nature of the disorder to the patients and offer suggestions regarding self-help.

5 Important rheumatological conditions

5.2 Osteoarthritis

Weight and exercise
Weight reduction probably does not influence outcome, but can reduce symptoms especially in symptomatic weight-bearing joints.

Patients should be encouraged to maintain activity, interspersed with rest during inflammatory exacerbations.

Physiotherapy
- Build up muscle strength.
- Increase range of motion.
- Pain relief and treatment of muscle spasm by using:
  ultrasound;
  diathermy;
  hot packs.
- Hydrotherapy — increases range of motion and muscle-strength whilst supporting body weight.
- Home exercises to be performed on a daily basis.

Aids
A walking stick can reduce the load through an osteoarthritic hip or knee by 30%. In severe disease, assessment by an occupational therapist may identify areas of specific need to maintain independence. Rubber heels on shoes reduce impact pressures on hip and knee.

Drugs (see also section 6.1)
- *Simple analgesic drugs* such as paracetamol should supplement the measures outlined above.
- *Non-steroidal anti-inflammatory agents* should be used for short-term treatment in inflammatory episodes.
- Local corticosteroids may be useful in the management of pericapsular and ligamentous areas of tenderness around joints.

5 Important rheumatological conditions

5.2 Osteoarthritis

Table 5.2. Secondary forms of OA

1 *Inflammatory states* (inflammatory joint disease associated with residual joint damage)
  (a) Healed rheumatoid arthritis
  (b) Healed Psoriatic arthropathy
  (c) Gout
  (d) Septic and tuberculous arthritis
  (e) Haemophilic arthropathy

2 *Endocrine diseases*
  (a) Acromegaly
  (b) Diabetes mellitus
  (c) Hypothyroidism

3 *Metabolic disorders*
  (a) Haemachromatosis
  (b) Ochronosis
  (c) Mucopolysaccharidoses
  (d) Wilson's disease

4 *Developmental disorders*
  (a) Legg–Calvé–Perthes disease
  (b) Slipped femoral epiphysis
  (c) Spondylo and multiple epiphyseal dysplasias
  (d) Hip dysplasias
  (e) Protrusio acetabuli

5 *Physical factors*
  (a) Avascular necrosis
  (b) Trauma — fractures through the joint
  (c) Meniscectomy
  (d) Neuropathic arthropathy
  (e) Long leg arthropathy
  (f) Joint laxity

Treatment of specific joints

Hands
Despite marked deformity, the hands usually function well. Intra-articular steroids are beneficial for painful thumb base OA. Rarely, arthroplasty or excision on this joint is needed.

5 Important rheumatological conditions

5.2 Osteoarthritis

Hip and knee
A walking stick is helpful. Total joint replacement has revolutionized treatment of severe OA hip (see section 6.3). Severe knee disease can be treated by osteotomy or prosthetic replacement.

Spine
See section 4.1.

OA of the feet
Local corticosteroid injection relieves pain due to inflammation of the 1st MTP. Hallux rigidus requires low-heeled shoes with firm soles, preferably fitted with metatarsal bars.

Prognosis
This is variable. Not all OA ends in joint replacement, and in some cases a severely affected joint may apparently heal with a reduction in symptoms.

Concentric hip disease has a better prognosis than superiolateral disease. The onset of OA in the very old may have a better outcome; however, a rapidly destructive variant associated with calcium hydroxyapatite cyrstals has been described in elderly females (section 5.5).

5 Important rheumatological conditions

5.3 Seronegative spondylarthropathies

5.3 Seronegative spondylarthropathies

These are an interrelated set of conditions and share several common features:
1 Negative tests for rheumatoid factor.
2 Inflammatory peripheral arthritis.
3 Radiographic sacroiliitis.
4 Clinical overlap.
5 Tendency to familial aggregation.

Included in this group of diseases are:
ankylosing spondylitis;
psoriatic arthropathy;
Reiter's syndrome;
reactive arthritis;
enteropathic arthropathy.

Some patients fulfil none of the accepted criteria for specific conditions and are designated as having an undifferentiated spondylarthropathy.

Ankylosing spondylitis (AS)
This is an inflammatory arthritis affecting the spine and sacroiliac joints. Thirty-five per cent of AS patients develop a peripheral arthritis which usually affects the lower limbs only.

Aetiology

Genetic. HLA B27 is present in:
95% of patients with AS;
50% of first degree relatives;
7% of the Caucasian population.

Environmental. In people possessing HLA B27, 20% at most show evidence of AS on X-ray (many are asymptomatic). Therefore, an additional environmental factor is involved. Interest is currently directed towards gut-derived bacterial antigens.

5 Important rheumatological conditions

5.3 Seronegative spondylarthropathies

Clinical features
1 Prevalence: 0.5%; males predominate 7:3.
2 Low back pain and stiffness — worse on waking and eases with exercise.
3 Chest pain — pain over costochondral junctions and manubriosternal and sternoclavicular joints.
4 Peripheral arthritis:
   more common in women;
   usually assymetric;
   hips, knees and shoulders common;
   small joints of hands and feet rare.
5 Enthesitis:
   plantar fasciitis;
   pelvic and chest wall tendon insertions.
6 Systemic:
   fever and weight loss.

Routine measurements include:
1 Chest expansion (normal is >5 cm).
2 Finger to floor distance.
3 Tragus to wall distance.
4 Schober's test (see section 1.2).

Complications
1 *Iritis*. Anterior uveitis occurs in 20% of patients.
2 *Cardiovascular disease*. Aortitis occurs in 3–5% and leads to aortic incompetence. Cardiac arrhythmias include complete heart block.
3 *Respiratory disease*. Reduced lung volume due to restriction of thoracic cage by costovertebral joint ankylosis. Patients compensate by increasing diaphragmatic excursion. Apical fibrosis and calcification and/or cavitation. Secondary infection with *Aspergillus fumigatus* may occur.
4 *Neurological complications*. Atlanto-axial subluxation may compromise the spinal cord. Fractures with little trauma may occur in the brittle rigid spine, most commonly in the cervical

5 Important rheumatological conditions

5.3 Seronegative spondylarthropathies

region. Quadriplegia may result and has a high mortality. Cauda equina syndrome — buttock or leg pain, bladder or bowel disturbance and variable sensory loss. Myelography usually reveals lumbar arachnoid diverticulae.

5 *Secondary amyloidosis* (AA amyloid). This complication is seen more frequently in juvenile AS and may cause death.

Differential diagnosis
The following six features should suggest the diagnosis of AS and distinguish it from other causes of back pain.
1 Age of onset <30 years.
2 Insidious onset.
3 Low back pain for more than 3 months.
4 Morning and rest stiffness.
5 Improvement with exercise.
6 Good response to NSAIDs.

Investigations
1 ESR, plasma viscosity and CRP: Usually elevated in active disease, but can be normal.
2 FBC: mild normochromic/cytic anaemia in severe disease.
3 HLA B27: casts doubt on diagnosis if negative.
4 X-rays (see Figs 5.6–5.8)
 (a) (SIJ): changes of sacro-iliitis are the earliest to appear, but may be delayed 2–3 years after onset of symptoms
 early: loss of definition of lower 2/3 joint space
 later: joint space narrowing, sclerosis and bony bridging of upper 1/3
 late: joint ankylosis with surrounding osteoporosis;
 (b) Spine: 'squaring' of vertebral body, erosion of anterior corners at insertion of annulus fibrosis ('Romanus lesion'), symmetrical syndesmophytes, thin vertical bony bridges originating from vertebral body angle, late disease produces the rigid 'bamboo spine';

5 Important rheumatological conditions

5.3 Seronegative spondylarthropathies

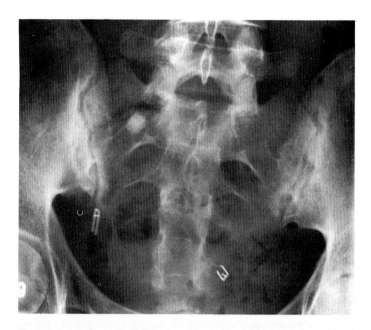

Fig. 5.6 Ankylosing spondylitis — early bilateral erosive sacroiliitis in a female showing poor definition of articular surfaces, focal erosion and ill-defined sclerosis. The left hip is abnormal.

(c) Pelvis: periostitis in the form of fluffy new bone formation at entheses.

Sacroiliitis should be differentiated from osteitis condensans ilii (multiparous women, asymptomatic X-ray finding of sclerosis affecting iliac bones adjacent to normal SIJs).

Syndesmophytes should be differentiated from:
1 Osteophytes: horizontal asymmetric bony outgrowths seen with disc space narrowing.
2 Ankylosing hyperostosis: large, beak-like bony outgrowths originating from the middle of the vertebral body, predominantly on left side.

5 Important rheumatological conditions

5.3 Seronegative spondylarthropathies

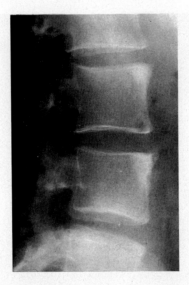

Fig. 5.7 Ankylosing spondylitis — active spine disease showing syndesmophyte formation and focal sclerosis with adjacent erosion at the surface of the enthesis (Romanus lesion) causing squaring of the vertebral body.

Management
1 *Pain relief* is usually obtained by NSAIDs (see section 6.1). Slow release indomethacin is very effective, whilst phenylbutazone is available for consultant-supervised prescription to those not responding to other NSAIDs.
2 *Local corticosteroids.* Intra-articular or peri-lesional injections of depot corticosteroids such as triamcinalone are useful for acutely inflamed joints and troublesome enthesitis.
3 *Smoking is emphatically discouraged* in view of the restriction of lung function.
4 *Exercise.* Regular daily exercise is important, but pain must first be relieved. Correct posture, particularly in bed, is advised —

5 Important rheumatological conditions

5.3 Seronegative spondylarthropathies

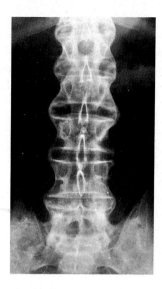

Fig. 5.8 Ankylosing spondylitis — end stage disease showing bony ankylosis of the sacro-ilial joints and extensive vertebral syndesmophytes (bamboo spine).

a firm mattress and only one pillow. Walking, swimming and jogging maintain fitness and joint mobility. Spinal exercises are useful.

5 *Physiotherapy* for specific measures to increase mobility and for supervision of an appropriate exercise regime that should be incorporated into the patient's daily routine.

6 *Education*. Information booklets for patients are produced by the ARC. Support is obtainable through a local branch of the National Ankylosing Spondylitis Society (NASS — see Appendix 1).

7 *Surgery*. Total hip replacement is most common. Cervical and lumbar osteotomies correct posture, stabilization of atlanto-axial subluxation, and condylar resection is available for ankylosis of the temporomandibular joint.

5 Important rheumatological conditions

5.3 Seronegative spondylarthropathies

8 *Radiotherapy.* Total spinal irradiation was used in the past but is associated with an excess mortality from leukaemia, aplastic anaemia and cancer. Local treatment is still occasionally used for localized inflammatory disease when other treatments have failed.

Disease course
Highly variable with spontaneous exacerbations and remissions. Often mild and self-limiting. After 20 years of disease, 65–80% of patients are still able to work full-time.

Psoriatic arthropathy
Only 5–7% of patients with psoriasis develop psoriatic arthritis, an inflammatory seronegative arthritis. Psoriasis affects 1–2% of the general population.

Aetiology: genetic factors involved

HLA B13, B17, Bw38	increased risk of developing psoriasis
HLA B27	psoriasis alone, 5–10%
	psoriatic arthropathy without sacroiliitis, 20%
	with sacroiliitis, 50–60%

Family history of psoriasis in 30%.

Clinical features
- Sex ratio equal.
- Psoriatic skin lesions develop at 20–30 years;
  arthritis develops within months to years;
  10% arthritis and skin lesions appear together;
  < 10% psoriatic arthritis 'sine psoriasis' — many go on to develop skin lesions later.
- Five patterns of arthropathy recognized.
  (a) DIP joint inflammation with nail involvement 10%;

5 Important rheumatological conditions

5.3 Seronegative spondylarthropathies

   (b) arthritis mutilans (5%). Deformity due to osteolysis of articulating ends of phalanges, metacarpals and metatarsals and sometimes large joints. 'Main en lorgnette' or 'opera glass hands' seen;

   (c) symmetrical polyarthritis very similar to RA except:
seronegative
no nodules
'sausage' digits (swollen, tender digit caused by a combination of joint and tendon sheath swelling); often similar changes in the feet;

   (d) monarthritis or asymmetrical oligoarthritis (70%). Often two or three DIP, PIP or MCP joints involved and there is flexor tenosynovitis.

   (e) ankylosing spondylitis with psoriasis (15%). Sacro-iliac and spinal involvement sometimes asymmetrical.

- Skin lesions. A thorough examination is required, especially 'hidden sites' — scalp, umbilicus, natal cleft.
- Nail changes. Pitting, ridging, and onicholysis.
- Other extra-articular features:
iritis 7%;
conjunctivitis 20%;
aortitis rare.

Investigations

Laboratory findings are non-specific. A raised serum urate in 10–20%, reflecting increased cell turnover.

The following changes can be seen in X-rays (Fig. 5.9).

- Asymmetrical joint involvement.
- Erosive changes at DIPs with relative sparing of the MCPs.
- Periosteal new bone formation.
- Joint ankylosis.
- Whittling of bone ends producing the pencil-in-cup deformity of IP joints.
- Findings in the axial skeleton of paravertebral ossification

5 Important rheumatological conditions

5.3 Seronegative spondylarthropathies

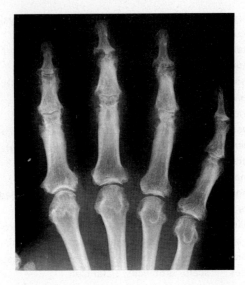

Fig. 5.9 Psoriatic arthritis showing involvement of the PIP and DIP joints, and proliferative periarticular erosions.

(rare), atypical and asymmetrical syndesmophytes, sacroiliitis — may be asymmetrical.

Management
1 Patients with spinal disease treated much as AS.
2 NSAIDs are effective in the majority.
3 Intra-articular or tendon sheath injections may be useful.
4 'Second-line agents' include:
   gold;
   azathioprine;
   methotrexate (see section 6.1);
   avoid antimalarials and systemic corticosteroids.
5 Surgery may be complicated by postoperative periarticular fibrosis and restriction of mobilization.
6 Treatment of psoriatic skin lesions (keratolytics, low dose

5 Important rheumatological conditions

5.3 Seronegative spondylarthropathies

topical corticosteroids, PUVA, retinoids, 1,25 cholecalciferol locally).

Reiter's syndrome
A syndrome comprising the classical triad of urethritis, conjunctivitis and arthritis.

Aetiology
1 *Infective*. It is a post infectious syndrome or 'reactive arthritis':
  (a) postdysenteric following infection with:
      Shigella flexneri or *dysenteriae*;
      Salmonella;
      Yersinia enterocolitica;
      Campylobacter jejuni;
  (b) post venereal, possibly associated with:
      Chlamydia trachomatis;
      Mycoplasma urea.
2 *Genetic*. 80% have HLA B27 antigen and 20% of B27 positive individuals who contract *Shigella* or *Salmonella* dysentery will develop Reiter's syndrome.

Clinical features
Predominantly males (15:1) although under-diagnosed in females, due to difficulty in diagnosing cervicitis and urethritis. Postdysenteric form develops after 1–3 weeks.
- *Arthritis*: inflammatory mono or asymmetrical oligoarthritis with the following distribution:
    predominantly affects the weight-bearing joints of the lower limbs;
    knees, ankles and IP joints of feet;
    sausage toe (dactylitis) is common;
    periostitis and enthesitis are characteristic;
    heel pain caused by Achilles tendinitis and plantar fasciitis;
    sacroiliitis (20%);
    ankylosing spondylitis (5%).

5 Important rheumatological conditions

5.3 Seronegative spondylarthropathies

- *Urethritis*. Usually clear, sterile urethral discharge (gleet) with minimal dysuria or systemic features.
- *Eye involvement*. Conjunctivitis, often transient, may lead to episcleritis, keratitis and corneal ulceration. Acute anterior uveitis occurs in 30%.
- *Mucocutaneous lesions*:

    painless mouth ulcers (27%) occur on palate, tongue and mucosa of cheeks;

    circinate balanitis (46%) in both postvenereal and postdysenteric forms;

    keratoderma blenorrhagica (22%) begins on feet and may involve palms;

Lesions begin as brown macules and progress to:

    papulovesicles and pustules;

    nail dystrophy and subungual hyperkeratosis.

- *Other lesions* are rare:

    pericarditis;

    aortitis;

    conduction abnormalities;

    pleurisy;

    transient pulmonary infiltrates;

    amyloidosis.

Investigations

1 ESR and viscosity are elevated during the acute phase.
2 Neutrophilia, mild hypochromic or normochromic anaemia.
3 X-rays:

    normal in early disease;

    later juxta-articular osteoporosis, joint space narrowing, erosions;

    periostitis such as calcaneal spurs;

    asymmetrical sacroiliitis;

    syndesmophytes with 'skip lesions'.

5 Important rheumatological conditions

5.3 Seronegative spondylarthropathies

Management
1 NSAIDs.
2 Intra-articular and perilesional depot corticosteroids.
3 Physiotherapy.
4 Education: use of condom and avoidance of multiple sexual partners advisable.
5 Watch for complications: uveitis, cardiovascular.
6 Severe disease: azathioprine, methotrexate.

Disease course
At 5 years the majority of patients have continuing disease with polyarthritis (80%), urethritis/cervicitis (40%), eye disease (30%), balanitis and mouth ulcers (25%) and 25% are unemployable or forced to change occupation.

Reactive arthritis due to *Yersinia*
Infections due to *Yersinia enterocolitica* are most often found in Scandinavia, Northern Europe, Canada and Japan.

Clinical features
1 Polyarthritis occurs 4–10 days after a mild diarrhoeal illness accompanied by:
   abdominal pain and fever;
   arthritis is usually additive not migratory, knees and ankles most commonly affected;
   arthritis is self-limiting after 1–4 months.
2 Fever, tendinitis and erythema nodosum may occur.

Investigations
Raised serum titre of anti-*Yersinia* antibodies.

Management
1 NSAIDs.
2 Intra-articular depot steroids.
3 Antibiotics are not useful for self-limiting arthritis.

5 Important rheumatological conditions

5.3 Seronegative spondylarthropathies

4 Septicaemia or septic arthritis can be treated by gentamycin or chloramphenicol.

Enteropathic arthritis

Inflammatory bowel disease

Clinical features
1 *Peripheral arthritis* occurs in 10–20%:
sex-incidence equal;
no increased frequency of HLA B27;
arthritis more common with extensive colitis;
oligoarthritis affecting knee, ankle, elbow and PIP finger joints;
activity of arthritis parallels activity of bowel disease in ulcerative colitis but not in Crohn's disease.
2 *Spondylitis* occurs in 4–5%:
males predominate;
70% have HLA B27;
may develop before or after onset of ulcerative colitis (UC);
unrelated to bowel disease.
3 Associated with erythema nodosum in UC.

Investigations
1 ESR, viscosity and CRP raised.
2 Microcytic, hypochromic anaemia.
3 Stool cultures in an exacerbation.
4 X-rays:
peripheral disease typically produces no residual deformity;
spondylitis identical to AS.

Management
1 Treatment of the colitis improves the peripheral arthritis, particularly in UC.
2 Sulphasalazine.
3 Corticosteroids.

5 Important rheumatological conditions

5.3 Seronegative spondylarthropathies

4 Colectomy in severe ulcerative colitis.
5 Caution should be taken with NSAIDs as they may worsen the bowel disease.
6 Intra-articular steroids may be useful.
  Treatment of the spondylitis follows that of ankylosing spondylitis.

Whipple's disease
Although rare, it is important to diagnose as will respond to specific therapy.

Aetiology
Associated with the presence of bacilli in PAS positive foamy macrophages seen in lymph nodes and the lamina propria of the small intestine. Similar organisms have been demonstrated in synovial biopsies.

Clinical features
1 Males predominate, 25–75 years.
2 Arthralgias or arthritis may occur up to 15 years before other clinical features:
  most often migratory, affecting knees and ankles;
  joint effusions may be present;
  residual deformity uncommon.
3 Other features:
  weight loss;
  fever;
  skin pigmentation;
  abdominal pain;
  steatorrhoea;
  lymphadenopathy;
  pericarditis;
  myopathy;
  diffuse neurological and eye abnormalities.

5 Important rheumatological conditions

5.3 Seronegative spondylarthropathies

Investigations
1 Anaemia.
2 Evidence of malabsorption:
 low folate;
 raised beta-carotenoids;
 increased faecal fat excretion.
3 Jejunal biopsy shows PAS positive foamy macrophages.
4 X-rays of joints usually normal.

Management
Tetracycline 250 mg q.d.s. for 1 year followed by cautious withdrawal. Short-term oral corticosteroids for initial control (3–4 weeks).

5 Important rheumatological conditions

5.4 Connective tissue diseases

5.4 Connective tissue diseases

Systemic lupus erythematosus (SLE)

Aetiology
The cause of SLE is unknown. The current hypothesis suggests a combination of infection and an abnormal host response.

Pathogenesis
- Circulating immune complexes probably initiate tissue damage in SLE. These complexes consist mainly of DNA and anti-DNA antibodies.
- Lymphocytotoxins which are toxic for T lymphocytes can be demonstrated in cryoprecipitates in patients with active SLE.

Prevalence
In Caucasian populations the prevalence is 1 in 2000. Increased prevalence is found amongst the black female population of San Francisco and the West Indies. Other areas with increased prevalence include Hong Kong, Singapore and China.

Clinical features
There is a striking female preponderance (9:1) with onset at any age, usually 20–40 years. In most patients the disease is mild, with arthralgia or arthritis occurring in 90%. Malaise, depression, pleuritic chest pain and fever are common in active disease.

The skin and mucous membranes
- Photosensitive rashes are very common, especially diffuse maculo-papular rashes. The classical 'butterfly rash' is seen in less than 50%.
- A small vessel vasculitis is common in the skin and affects the hands, forearms and elbows.
- Livido reticularis.
- Raynaud's phenomenon.

5 Important rheumatological conditions

5.4 Connective tissue diseases

- Alopecia occurs in 65% and is often a good clinical guide to disease activity.
- Mouth ulcers.

Musculoskeletal system
- The chronic polyarthritis of SLE is typically symmetrical, non-deforming and non-erosive. Flexor tenosynovitis is common, tendon contractures are occasionally seen and a deforming arthritis (Jaccoud's arthropathy) is seen in a few patients.
- Aseptic necrosis most commonly affecting the hip may occur either due to the disease or secondary to corticosteroids.
- Myositis may be seen.

CNS disease
- CNS lupus can involve the whole spectrum of neurological disease including chorea, cranial nerve palsies, migraine, convulsions and spinal cord lesions.
- Retinal involvement can be visualized as cytoid bodies.

The kidneys
- Clinically significant renal disease is seen in a minority of patients, although all patients with SLE probably have minor histological abnormalities.
- Nocturia, hypertension, oedema and proteinuria may occur together with progressive renal failure.

The lungs
- Pulmonary manifestations include atelactasis, pneumonitis and 'shrinking lungs' with rising diaphragms.

Other features
- Polyserositis occurs in 50%. Pleurisy is more common than pericarditis and sterile peritonitis occurs infrequently.
- Splenomegaly, lymphadenopathy and anaemia are common.

There may be a history of recurrent abortions and thrombosis in those possessing the lupus anticoagulant.

5 Important rheumatological conditions

5.4 Connective tissue diseases

Investigations

1 Urinalysis: proteinuria and/or haematuria requires the examination of a fresh specimen of urine. Red cell or white cell casts indicate active renal disease. Infection should be excluded.

2 Full blood count: a normochromic, normocytic anaemia is common as is lymphopenia. An immune thrombocytopenia and haemolytic anaemia (Coombs positive) can occur.

3 Urea and electrolytes, creatinine clearance to determine renal function.

4 Clotting studies: the APTT is prolonged in those with lupus anticoagulant.

5 Complement levels may be low in active disease. In addition, deficiency of early complement components predisposes to SLE.

6 Autoantibody tests: a large variety of antinuclear antibodies have been defined (see Table 2.3) and have occasional clinical relevance. Anti-double-stranded DNA antibodies are specific for SLE, although not always present, and can be useful in monitoring disease activity in the individual patient. Cryoprecipitates occur in 60%.

7 Biopsy of clinically unaffected skin demonstrates immune complexes at the dermal–epidermal junction ('lupus band test').

Management

General principles
The patient in remission requires no therapy, even if laboratory tests are abnormal, such as an elevated DNA binding value. Patients with abnormal laboratory tests but clinically inactive SLE require careful observation. Treatment should match the clinical activity of SLE, which is very variable.

1 Avoidance of events known to precipitate exacerbations, such as ultraviolet light exposure, infections and drugs (see p. 141), is important. Strong ultraviolet barrier creams are available.

2 Non-steroidal anti-inflammatory drugs (NSAIDs) for arthritis, arthralgia, tendinitis and mild systemic involvement.

5 Important rheumatological conditions

5.4 Connective tissue diseases

3 Hydroxychloroquine (200–400 mg/day) is useful for photosensitivity, cutaneous lesions, mild constitutional symptoms, arthralgia and arthritis. Ocular toxicity is low (see Chapter 6).
4 Corticosteroids. Fever, skin involvement, arthritis or serositis may require corticosteroids to suppress activity. Low dose therapy (< 15 mg prednisolone) in a single daily dose is usually sufficient. For patients with major organ involvement (heart, kidney, central nervous system), myositis and haematological crises (haemolysis, thrombocytopenia), high dose corticosteroids are indicated. The starting dose is 1 mg/kg/day of prednisolone.
5 Plasmapheresis helps the rash but not the systemic manifestations.

CNS lupus
Exclude infection as a cause of CNS involvement in SLE. In CNS lupus, CSF studies are normal, glucose may be low. EEG changes in 50%. Angiography and CT scans are of little help except to exclude a cerebral abscess.

The majority of patients with CNS lupus can be managed with the introduction or elevation of corticosteroid dosage to 40–60 mg/day of prednisolone, together with intravenous cyclophosphamide 500 mg.

Anticonvulsants for seizures and psychotropic drugs for psychoses and behavioural disorders may be needed.

Lupus nephritis
Clinical renal disease means increased morbidity and mortality. Hypertension and urinary tract infections should be treated vigorously.

Corticosteroids are beneficial (> 1 mg/kg/day) for active nephritis and should be continued until there is clearing of the urinary sediment.

The addition of azathioprine (2 mg/kg) or cyclophosphamide (100–150 mg/day) confers added advantage over corticosteroids

5 Important rheumatological conditions

5.4 Connective tissue diseases

alone and may have a corticosteroid-sparing effect.

Pulmonary lupus
Secondary bacterial infection is common in lupus pneumonitis. Give appropriate antibiotic as well as corticosteroid.

Drug-induced lupus
A number of drugs are known to induce SLE. Amongst the most common are:
- Hydralazine.
- Procainamide.
- Isoniazid.
- Phenytoin.
- Chlorpromazine.

Predisposing factors include:
- Old age.
- Slow acetylator status.
- HLA DR4 (for hydralazine).

Clinical features are similar to idiopathic disease although renal involvement is rare. Investigations show high titre ANA which is predominantly anti-histone. Anti-dsDNA is present in only 10%. Rapid resolution follows discontinuation of the drug.

Lupus in pregnancy
- Lupus does not impair fertility unless disease is severe although there is increased maternal morbidity and foetal loss with active disease.
- Recurrent abortion is associated with presence of anticardiolipin antibody and correlates with placental vein thrombosis.
- Both delivery and abortion may be followed by disease flares.
- Patients should be advised against conception unless the disease has been in remission on less than 15 mg of prednisolone for 6 months or more both by clinical and serological parameters.

5 Important rheumatological conditions

5.4 Connective tissue diseases

- Patients should be monitored regularly throughout pregnancy and given steroids as necessary. Weekly platelet counts, complement levels and anti-DNA antibody levels are advisable during the third trimester. Corticosteroids should be increased to cover delivery.
- The contraceptive pill should probably be avoided as a first-line method of birth control.

Neonatal lupus
This condition is rare. Transient rashes, Coombs positive anaemia and congenital heart block are described.

There is a high prevalence of anti-Ro antibody and HLA DR3 in the mothers of affected infants.

Scleroderma (systemic sclerosis)

Aetiology
The cause is unknown.

Pathology
The small arteries show intimal proliferation, medial thinning and collagen cuffing that occurs around the adventitia and encases the artery. The lesion is best seen in the kidney and peripheral vasculature.

Clinical features
There is a female preponderance (3 : 1) usually in middle age. There are three clinical types.

1 CREST — an acronym denoting patients with:
  Calcinosis;
  Raynaud's;
  OEsophageal involvement;
  Sclerodactyly;
  Telangectasia.

5 Important rheumatological conditions

5.4 Connective tissue diseases

It is considered a benign variant, with a small incidence of systemic disease. It often remains static or progresses at a very slow rate. There is anti-centromere antibody in 60–90%. Some patients develop pulmonary hypertension.

2 Acrosclerosis — cutaneous involvement of the extremities:
   distal forearms;
   hands (finger contractures, pulp atrophy);
   feet;
   also around eyes (difficult eversion of the eyelids), mouth (microstomia and radial furrowing) and neck.

Raynaud's disease is prominent and may lead to ischaemic ulcers and gangrene. Abnormalities of the nailfold capillaries also develop.

The systemic sites involved are listed below.

- The gut:
  oesophageal dysfunction with dysphagia, vomiting and reflux common;
  malabsorption secondary to small bowel atrophy and bacterial overgrowth;

- The lungs:
  restrictive lung disease;
  pleural effusion;

- The heart:
  myocarditis;
  pericarditis;

- The kidneys:
  significant renal disease is rare in this group.

Some patients develop a proximal myositis.

3 Diffuse scleroderma
   skin involvement extends proximally on to the trunk;
   often rapidly progressive;
   Raynaud's disease is less common;

5 Important rheumatological conditions

5.4 Connective tissue diseases

calcinosis and telangiectasia infrequent;
systemic disease often severe and fulminant renal disease may occur.

Investigations
Laboratory tests:
  most inflammatory markers are normal;
  renal function should be assessed;
  antinuclear antibodies common;
  anti-Scl-70 often found in those with widespread cutaneous disease (see also Chapter 2).
X-ray tests of hands show (see Fig. 5.10):
  calcinosis;
  contractures;
  resorption of the end of the distal phalanx.
Barium studies may be used for dysphagia (barium swallow) and malabsorption (small bowel).
Respiratory function tests are often abnormal (reduced transfer factor).

Management
- Therapy is symptomatic and organ-specific.
- Raynaud's disease. Protection against the cold is required:
  heated gloves;
  calcium antagonists such as nifedipine (10 mg t.d.s.);
  prostaglandin E_1 for ischaemic crises.
- Reflux oesophagitis:
  antacids;
  H_2 antagonists;
  elevation of head of bed.
- Bowel bacterial overgrowth:
  tetracycline.
- Renal disease:
  control hypertension;
  captopril for renal crises.

5 Important rheumatological conditions

5.4 Connective tissue diseases

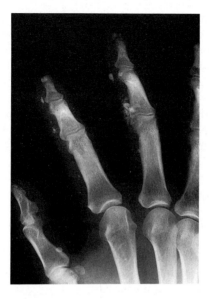

Fig. 5.10 Systemic sclerosis showing flexion deformities, tuft resorption and soft tissue calcification.

Specific treatment is disappointing. D-penicillamine and colchicine may improve cutaneous sclerosis in early disease, but have no effect on systemic involvement.

Eosinophilic fasciitis
This is a rare condition that may be initially confused with systemic sclerosis because of similar skin manifestions. It is distinguished by the absence of Raynaud's disease and lack of involvement of other systems. Blood and tissue eosinophilia are characteristic and histology demonstrates prominent involvement of the deeper tissues including the lower subcutis, fascia and muscle. The condition often responds to corticosteroids and the prognosis is good.

5 Important rheumatological conditions

5.4 Connective tissue diseases

Dermatomyositis, polymyositis
Polymyositis is an idiopathic, necrotizing inflammation of muscle. When this is associated with a distinctive rash (see below) it is termed dermatomyositis.

Aetiology
Cell mediated immunity (CMI) against patient's muscle cells is found. Cytotoxic lymphocytes are sometimes found in involved muscles. There is humoral antinuclear antibody (Jo-1).

Clinical features
These are rare conditions, with a female preponderance (3 : 1) and onset at any age including childhood.

Proximal muscle weakness is prominent leading to difficulty rising from a chair, ascending stairs or putting on a coat (when the shoulder girdle is involved).

Characteristic dermatological changes are:
lilac discoloration of the eyelids;
periorbital oedema;
scaly erythematous rash overlying extensor surfaces of MCPs, knees, elbows and medial malleoli;
nailfold capillary dilation;
'tissue paper atrophy' of skin over knuckles.

There is a significant association with malignancy in the older age groups, especially middle-aged males. There is no specific type of malignancy.

Investigations
1 Myometry.
2 Muscle enzymes (CPK, aldolase, AST).
3 EMG changes:
   short small polyphasic action potentials;
   fibrillation;
   positive sharp waves and insertional irritability.
4 Muscle biopsy: necrosis, phagocytosis, regeneration,

5 Important rheumatological conditions

5.4 Connective tissue diseases

perifascicular atrophy and inflammation.
5 Antibodies to Jo-1 (histidyl tRNA synthetase) in 20%.
6 Exhaustive tests for malignancy not warranted.

Management
1 High dose corticosteroids initially (prednisolone 60 mg/day). After 2 months, reduce dosage slowly providing muscle strength has improved.
2 Add methotrexate (7.5–15 mg weekly) or azathioprine (2 mg/kg/day) when muscle strength has not improved after 2 months with prednisolone.
3 Continue to monitor progress with muscle enzymes and repeated and careful assessment of muscle power (myometry).
4 Maintenance treatment, once remission has been achieved, should be continued for at least 2 years.
5 Hydroxychloroquine (200 mg b.d.) can be used in mild disease or to maintain remission.

Sjögren's syndrome (Sicca syndrome)

Two types are recognized:
  primary Sjögren's;
  secondary Sjögren's, which is associated with rheumatoid arthritis, systemic sclerosis or SLE.

Pathology
Salivary and lachrymal glandular tissue is infiltrated with lymphocytes and plasma cells.

Clinical features
- Age and sex: the primary type occurs in females over 50 years.
- Dryness of eyes and mouth (keratoconjunctivitis sicca) is the most common feature.
- Raynaud's phenomenon and recurrent parotitis are more common in primary Sjögren's syndrome.
- Kidneys: there is tubular dysfunction in 25% of patients with:

5 Important rheumatological conditions

5.4 Connective tissue diseases

  renal tubular acidosis;
  aminoaciduria;
  phosphaturia;
  a diabetes insipidus-like picture results from patient's compulsion to drink to relieve dry mouth and throat.
- Lungs: there is small airways obstruction with:
  interstitial lymphocyte infiltration;
  recurrent chest infections.
- CNS: there are cranial and peripheral neuropathies.

Investigations
- Schirmer's test (see section 1.2).
- Rose–Bengal staining/slit lamp examination of the cornea. minor salivary gland biopsy.
- ANF positive in 50%.
- Ro (SSA) 60%
  La (SSB) 36% } in primary type.

Treatment
Treatment is symptomatic.
- Hypromellose eye drops (artificial tears) should be used regularly.
- Surgery to block the lacrimal duct may help more severe cases.
- Avoid drugs known to contribute to xerostomia (see Table 5.3).
- Regular dental hygiene is essential to reduce dental caries.

Table 5.3. Classes of drug contributing to xerostomia

Antidepressants
Drugs used to treat Parkinson's disease
Antihypertensives (beta-blockers, diuretics)
Antispasmodics and anticholinergics
Antipsychotics

5 Important rheumatological conditions

5.4 Connective tissue diseases

- Xerostomia and dental hygiene may be helped with such products as Oral Balance Moisturising Gel, Biotene Dental Chewing Gum, Moi-Stir oral swabsticks.

Complications
Vasculitis occurs in 10% of patients.
 There is an increased risk of developing a lymphoproliferative malignancy. This may be heralded by:
 reduction in serum immunoglobulins;
 lymphadenopathy;
 splenomegaly.

Overlap syndromes
There is considerable overlap between the connective tissue disorders. Such patients present with features common to a number of diseases, but in time one pattern emerges. Such diseases are best termed 'overlap syndromes' or 'undifferentiated connective tissue disease' and their characteristics should be defined.

Mixed connective tissue disease (MCTD)
This condition has been defined serologically by high titres to nuclear ribonuclear protein (RNP). Clinical features were then collated and the resulting syndrome was termed 'mixed connective tissue disease'. It is now felt that these patients represent a sub-group of SLE. The clinical features in MCTD are:
 polyarthritis;
 Raynaud's phenomenon;
 swollen hands or sclerodactyly;
 reduced oesophageal motility;
 myositis;
 low incidence of clinical renal disease.
A good clinical response to corticosteroid therapy has been reported.

5.5 The crystal arthropathies

Gout

There are four stages of gout:

1 Asymptomatic hyperuricaemia: it may be many years before the first attack of gout occurs.
2 Acute gout is an inflammatory reaction to monosodium urate crystals.
3 Intercritical gout is the period between attacks.
4 Chronic tophaceous gout represents the gradual accumulation of crystal deposits (tophi) in joints and subcutaneous tissues, producing soft tissue and bony changes and deformity.

Aetiology

Gout invariably occurs in the context of hyperuricaemia. Hyperuricaemia may develop in three ways (Table 5.4):
  excessive production of uric acid;
  increased catabolism of nucleic acids;
  decreased excretion of uric acid.
Precipitating factors for an acute attack include:
  concurrent illness;
  trauma;
  over-indulgence in food or drink;
  surgery.

Clinical features

Males predominate (15:1), age 35–60 years, whilst the majority of female sufferers are postmenopausal.

Acute attack has an abrupt onset, often at night and very painful; there is marked joint and periarticular swelling with skin erythema — scaling occurs with resolution.

Moderate pyrexia is also common. Leucocytosis, raised ESR or plasma viscosity reflect the severity of the inflammation.

5 Important rheumatological conditions

5.5 The crystal arthropathies

Table 5.4. Causes of hyperuricaemia

1 *Excessive production of uric acid (uncommon)*
   Idiopathic
   Abnormalities of purine biosynthesis
   (a) enzyme deficiency: hypoxanthine guanine phosphoribosyl transferase (HGPRT), adenine phosphoribosyl transferase (APRT)
   (b) enzyme excess: 5 phosphoribosyl−1−pyrophosphate synthetase (PRPP)
   Von Gierke's glycogen storage disease (increased PRPP)
   Excessive dietary intake of proteins

2 *Excessive catabolism of nucleic acids (uncommon)*
   Myeloproliferative diseases
   Haemolysis
   Carcinomatosis
   Cytotoxic therapy
   Severe starvation
   Psoriasis
   Gaucher's disease
   Multiple myeloma

3 *Decreased renal excretion of uric acid (common)*
   Idiopathic
   Alcoholism
   Chronic renal failure
   Hyperparathyroidism
   Lactic acidosis
   Lead poisoning (saturnine gout)
   Diuretics and other drugs (see Table 5.6)
   Down's syndrome
   Myxoedema
   Berylliosis

Joints involved are:
1st MTP 70%;
elbow 7%;
ankle/foot 34%;
wrist 7%;
knee 20%;

5 Important rheumatological conditions

5.5 The crystal arthropathies

    finger 12%;
    other 17%;
In 6% of patients, gout is polyarticular; in 4% it is extra-articular.

In *tophaceous gout*, tophi occur in relation to joints, tendons or bursae, especially over bony prominences and pinna of ear. They are also described on vocal cords, aorta and heart valves. Elderly women on chronic diuretic therapy may develop tophaceous gout especially in the hand at sites with previous OA.

Gout is positively associated with:
    obesity;
    hypertension;
    hypertriglyceridaemia;
    cardiovascular disease;
    high alcohol intake;
    family history of gout.

The kidney
Renal involvement is an important complication of gout.
- Nephrolithiasis — 25% of gouty patients (both uric acid and calcium stones).
- Acute tubular necrosis due to deposition of uric acid crystals in the tubules. May be caused by aggressive chemotherapy for malignant disease without allopurinol cover.
- Proteinuria and impaired renal function may also occur and are probably a function of associated hypertension and renovascular disease.

Differential diagnosis
The acute attack is usually characteristic. However, attacks may be mild and occasionally polyarticular. Commonly confused states are:
    cellulitis;
    thrombophlebitis;
    septic arthritis;

5 Important rheumatological conditions

5.5 The crystal arthropathies

pseudogout.

In the hands chronic gout may superficially resemble rheumatoid arthritis.

Investigations

1 Examine joint fluid or tophus for negatively birefringent, needle-shaped crystals.

2 Hyperuricaemia: serum urate >0.42 mmol/l (males), >0.36 mmol/l (females). Note that serum urate may be normal if urate lowering therapy has already been instituted (e.g. large doses of aspirin).

3 Urea and electrolytes and creatinine clearance to detect renal involvement.

4 Spot urine sample for urinary urate/creatinine ratio: normal is <0.5, increased in over-producers.

5 Fasting triglycerides.

6 X-rays (Fig. 5.11):
early gout — non-specific appearances;
tophaceous gout — soft tissue masses; erosions, punched-out, well-defined with sclerotic, sometimes overhanging margins (Martel's hook); IVP — if stones suspected.

Management

In *acute attack*: NSAIDs, e.g. indomethacin 50 mg t.d.s. (does not affect serum urate level).

- Colchicine is used where NSAIDs are contraindicated. Initial dose 1 mg followed by 0.5 mg 2 hourly until the attack is controlled. No more should be given for 8 days as the half-life is very long. GI toxicity common after 5 mg; maximum dose 12 tablets/24 h.

Reduce dose in hepatic or renal insufficiency, in which colchicine has been associated with systemic toxicity including bone marrow suppression and neuropathy.

- Oral steroids may be used in severe unresponsive attacks.

5 Important rheumatological conditions

5.5 The crystal arthropathies

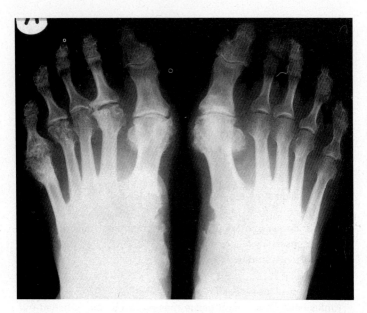

Fig. 5.11 Gout showing extensive bone proliferation at tendon insertions, well-defined erosions due to tophi and concomitant hypertrophic OA.

Exacerbations may occur on stopping therapy and can be prevented by NSAID cover.

In the *long-term*: identification and appropriate treatment of associated conditions such as hypertension and hyperlipidaemia.
- Dietary advice for obesity and avoidance of excessive intake of purine rich foods (Table 5.5) and alcohol.
- Avoidance or reduction of other risk factors, e.g. chronic diuretic usage in elderly females or the use of other uricostatic drugs (Table 5.6).

Indications for long-term treatment are:

5   Important rheumatological conditions

5.5   The crystal arthropathies

Table 5.5. Foods rich in purines

> Beer
> Sweetbreads
> Kidney
> Liver
> Brains
> Anchovies
> Sardines
> Yeast

Table 5.6. Uricosuric and uricostatic drugs

> *Uricosuric drugs*
> High doses of aspirin >4 g/day
> Sulphinpyrazone
> Probenacid
> Azapropazone
>
> *Uricostatic drugs*
> Pyrazinamide
> Thiazides
> Frusemide
> Ethacrinic acid
> Low doses of aspirin <4 g/day

frequent attacks of acute gout (more than two a year or more than 2 weeks off work);

chronic joint damage;

tophi;

evidence of renal damage or stones;

There are two main types of specific therapy available:

1 Uricosuric agents: probenecid 0.5–1 g (divided doses, max 3 g); sulphinpyrazone 100 mg t.d.s (max 800 mg divided doses); azapropazone 600 mg b.d. Note that the uricosuric action of these drugs is abolished by concomitant administration of salicylates.

5 Important rheumatological conditions

5.5 The crystal arthropathies

2 Xanthine oxidase inhibitor: allopurinol should be administered in a dose of 100 mg, increasing until control is achieved (usual dose 300 mg, max 800 mg). It is the drug of first choice in major overexcretors of uric acid, in those with renal insufficiency or with renal stones and in those receiving chemotherapy (prevention of acute uric acid nephropathy). Both uricosuric and xanthine oxidase drugs may be used concurrently in severe disease. See Table 5.7 for adverse effects.

Practical points

1 Apart from azapropazone, all long-term treatment should be preceded by colchicine or an NSAID and accompanied by a concomitant NSAID for at least a month to avoid an acute attack of gout as urate is mobilized.

2 Initiation of long-term uricosuric treatment should be accompanied by a high fluid intake to avoid uric acid deposition in the kidney.

3 Do not institute long-term treatment at the first attack of gout. It may be the sole attack or the only attack for some years. Hypouricaemic therapy is not without risk (Table 5.7).

4 Although gout sufferers invariably are hyperuricaemic, the converse is not true. Do not assume that joint pain in a hyperuricaemic subject is due to gout, unless more specific evidence is available.

5 Asymptomatic mild hyperuricaemia does not require drug treatment and usually responds to dietary and alcohol restriction.

Table 5.7. Adverse effects of hypouricaemic therapy

Allopurinol
In general, well tolerated and remarkably safe over many years of treatment. Adverse effects rare, but the following have been reported
(a) The skin
    (i) Pruritic rash 2% (increased to 20% with concomitant use of ampicillin)
    (ii) Allopurinol hypersensitivity syndrome (more common in renal or hepatic impairment)
        immune complex vasculitis

5 Important rheumatological conditions

5.5 The crystal arthropathies

Table 5.7. (cont.)

      eosinophilia
      hepatitis
      progressive renal failure
      arthralgia
  (iii) Exfoliative erythroderma
  (iv) Stevens–Johnson syndrome
  (v) Toxic epidermal necrolysis
(b) The gut
  (i) Nausea and vomiting
  (ii) Granulomatous hepatitis
(c) The blood
    Few reports of a decrease in the formed elements of the blood, usually with hepatic or renal impairment
(d) The kidney
    Xanthine stones may occur with prolonged therapy

Probenecid
(a) CNS
    Headache
    Dizziness
(b) The gut
    Nausea, vomiting, anorexia
(c) The blood
    Anaemia and haemolytic anaemia
(d) The skin
    Sore gums
    Flushing
    Hypersensitivity reactions
(e) Rarely
    Nephrotic syndrome
    Hepatic necrosis
    Aplastic anaemia

Sulphinpyrazone
(a) The skin
    Rash
(b) The gut
    GI bleeding has been reported
(c) The kidney
    Impairment of renal function with changes in electrolyte balance
(d) The blood
    Blood dyscrasias may occur at any time

5 Important rheumatological conditions

5.5 The crystal arthropathies

Calcium pyrophosphate deposition
Evidence of calcium pyrophosphate dihydrate crystals within the joint is associated with three different clinical conditions which, however, may show considerable overlap:
1 Radiological chondrocalcinosis — common, age related deposition of calcium pyrophosphate in articular cartilage, especially fibrocartilage, most commonly symptom-free.
2 Pyrophosphate arthropathy — chronic or sub-acute.
3 Acute pseudogout (acute crystal arthropathy).

Aetiology
Predisposing factors are listed below.
- Age: there is a rising prevalence with age.
- Familial: familial forms of chondrocalcinosis have been documented. Probably, it is autosomal dominant.
- Metabolic:
  hyperparathyroidism;
  haemochromatosis;
  hypothyroidism;
  gout;
  ochronosis;
  Wilson's disease;
  amyloidosis;
  hypomagnesaemia;
  hypophosphatasia.
- Traumatic:
  joint laxity;
  trauma, e.g. meniscectomy.
- Other: osteochondromatosis.

Clinical features

Radiological chondrocalcinosis
- Prevalence rare <60 years, occurs in 40% of those aged 90.

5 Important rheumatological conditions

5.5 The crystal arthropathies

- Often asymptomatic.
- May be associated with symptoms of OA, acute pseudogout or pyrophosphate arthropathy.

Clinical pyrophosphate arthropathy
- Often indistinguishable from other forms of OA. Some patients may be differentiated on the basis of:
  joint distribution — wrist, shoulder common but rare in OA;
  joint effusions may be large and troublesome;
  marked deformity: 10% have a destructive form of the disease;
  radiographic findings (see below).

Pseudogout
- Male predominance, 2:1.
- Acute episode of inflammatory arthritis.
- Pyrexia.
- May be distinguished from gout by:
  onset less acute;
  different joint distribution: knee (80%), hand/wrist (35%), ankle (15%), polyarticular (20%);
  attacks less severe, last longer;
  patients older, more often female;
  synovial fluid examination.
- Attacks may be precipitated by intercurrent disease and trauma, especially surgery.

Differential diagnosis:

Acute pseudogout may be confused with:
  septic arthritis;
  rheumatoid arthritis;
  periarthritis — deposits in tendon insertions, especially quadriceps and achilles;
  haemarthrosis — effusions may be blood-stained.

5 Important rheumatological conditions

5.5 The crystal arthropathies

Investigations
Synovial fluid examination demonstrates positively birefringent, oblong crystals.

In young patients a predisposing factor should be sought including screening for metabolic disease.

Radiology (Figs 5.12, 5.13):
- Chondrocalcinosis, a thin line of calcification, is most commonly seen at:
   menisci of the knee;
   triangular ligament of the wrist;
   pubic symphysis;
   labra of shoulder and hip.
- Pyrophosphate arthropathy resembles a hypertrophic form of OA with:
   exuberant osteophytosis;
   loose bodies;

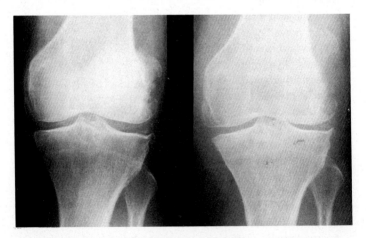

Fig. 5.12 Chondrocalcinosis showing linear calcification of the fibrocartilage of the knee. Note subsequent shedding of crystals and loss of cartilage width.

5 Important rheumatological conditions

5.5 The crystal arthropathies

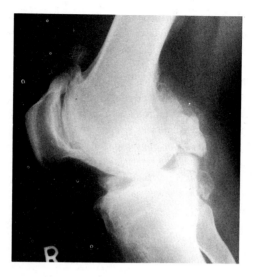

Fig. 5.13 Pyrophosphate arthropathy giving a 'hypertrophic OA' picture showing florid osteophytosis, marked patello-femoral disease and loose bodies.

  chondrocalcinosis;
  large sub-articular cysts;
  marked patello-femoral disease.
- Acute pseudogout usually shows evidence of chondrocalcinosis or pyrophosphate arthropathy.

Management
- *Asymptomatic chondrocalcinosis* requires no intervention.
- *Acute pseudogout* is treated with NSAIDs or intra-articular injection of 25 mg of triamcinolone acetonide if sepsis excluded. Colchicine 0.6 mg b.d. may help control recurrent attacks.
- *Pyrophosphate arthropathy* is treated along the same lines as OA (see section 5.2).

Large, recurrent joint effusions not responding to intra-articular steroids may benefit from the use of radioactive colloids such as ^{90}yttrium.

Calcium hydroxyapatite
Crystals of calcium hydroxyapatite comprise the main mineral component of bone. They may also be identified in joint fluids, most commonly in patients with osteoarthritis and in periarticular deposits. They are associated with two clinical conditions.

Calcific tendinitis and peritendinitis

Aetiology
Acute inflammatory reaction following the release of minute crystals from calcified tendinous deposit.

Clinical features
- Occurs in the younger age groups including children.
- Abrupt onset of severe pain.
- Effusion sometimes present (shoulder).
- Occasionally recurrent attacks in multiple sites.
- Any tendon may be affected:
  commonest in rotator cuff tendons in the shoulder;
  also around greater trochanter;
  medial ligament of knee (Peligrini—Stieda disease).

Investigations
X-ray will show deposit as dense discrete shadows (Fig. 5.14) which, once ruptured, becomes a diffuse cloud of calcification surrounding the original area.

Treatment
1 Strong analgesics in the acute phase, followed by NSAIDs.
2 Local corticosteroid injections can exacerbate the pain.
3 Small deposits may be aspirated through a wide bore needle.

5 Important rheumatological conditions

5.5 The crystal arthropathies

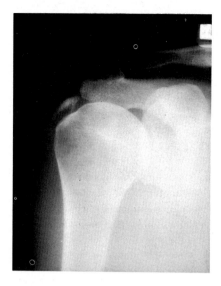

Fig. 5.14 Calcific periarthritis showing radiodense opacity overlying the superolateral aspect of the humerus.

4 Large deposits may require surgical removal.

Idiopathic destructive arthritis (Milwaukee shoulder, cuff tear arthropathy, apatite-associated destructive arthritis)
This is a destructive arthritis associated with large amounts of hydroxyapatite crystals in the synovial fluid.

Clinical features
- Usually elderly women.
- Voluminous blood-stained effusions.
- Shoulder most commonly affected.
- Also hip, knee and talocrural.
- No other cause for arthropathy.

5 Important rheumatological conditions

5.5 The crystal arthropathies

Investigations
1 Blood tests normal including plasma viscosity, CRP, rheumatoid factor.
2 Synovial fluid for hydroxyapatite crystals. Cell count normal.
3 X-rays show soft tissue swelling:
   marked bony attrition;
   subchondral sclerosis;
   loose bodies.

Treatment
1 Symptomatic — analgesics, physiotherapy.
2 Surgical — joint replacement may be difficult.
Treatment of other complications, such as pressure on the brachial plexus from a dislocated humeral head.

5 Important rheumatological conditions

5.6 Polymyalgia rheumatica and giant cell arteritis

5.6 Polymyalgia rheumatica and giant cell arteritis

Polymyalgia rheumatica (PMR)
PMR is a treatable, disabling condition of the elderly of unknown aetiology. A proportion of patients develop giant cell (temporal) arteritis (GCA) with its risks of blindness. PMR must be distinguished from other conditions, especially malignancy, that may present in a similar fashion.

Aetiology
Unknown: no infectious agent has been identified. Investigation of painful muscle has proved unhelpful. Raised levels of anticardiolipin antibodies (ACL) and disappearance of lymphocyte expression of CD 8 markers have been found in some patients with GCA.

Clinical features
- Sex ratio mirrors community; affects those over 60 years.
- Muscular pain and stiffness:
  often abrupt onset;
  shoulder and hip girdles principally affected;
  may be asymmetric initially.
- Muscle tenderness.
- Restricted shoulder movement in 90% at onset.
- Transient, non-deforming synovitis, 20%
- May present as shoulder–hand syndrome.

Differential diagnosis
1 Diseases with raised ESR or plasma viscosity:
   (a) prodromal phase of RA, or other connective tissue disease;
   (b) thyrotoxic myopathy;
   (c) occult TB;
   (d) multiple myeloma;
   (e) occult cancer;
   (f) carcinomatous neuromyopathy.

5   Important rheumatological conditions

5.6   Polymyalgia rheumatica and giant cell arteritis

2 ESR or plasma viscosity normal:
   (a) Parkinsonism;
   (b) hypothyroidism;
   (c) osteomalacia;
   (d) polycythaemia.

Investigations
No specific test, mainly to exclude other diagnoses.
1 ESR often >100 mm/h.
2 FBC — normochromic, normocytic anaemia common, rarely severe.
3 Liver function tests.
4 Calcium studies.
5 Thyroid function tests.
6 Serum immunoglobulins and electrophoretic strip.
7 Rheumatoid factor.
8 CXR and hands and feet if appropriate.

Management
The correct diagnosis is essential as the treatment is long-term, may mask other conditions and has possible adverse effects. Don't rush into treatment unless you suspect giant cell arteritis.
1 *Prednisolone*. The response is rapid and often dramatic compared with the partial or absent response to NSAIDs. A therapeutic test which helps confirm the diagnosis is 'the steroid sandwich'. Weeks 1 and 3: placebo tablets (ascorbic acid 50 mg b.d.) are given; week 2 prednisolone 5 mg b.d. is given. The patient is not informed which tablet is which, but that treatment is being tried with hormones and vitamins. The patient keeps a diary of symptoms, which should then confirm the positive response to corticosteroids and the return of symptoms in the third week. Thereafter treatment is adjusted up or down in 1 mg steps according to need. Regular follow-up is required with monitoring of symptoms and ESR. Few patients require more

5 Important rheumatological conditions

5.6 Polymyalgia rheumatica and giant cell arteritis

than 10 mg per day. Most have a critical level between 5 and 10 mg, below which symptoms return.

2 *Injections of corticosteroids* into the subacromial bursa may prove useful if shoulder stiffness is the main problem.

3 *Azathioprine* 50 mg b.d. can be used as a steroid sparing agent in the very few patients where high and potentially toxic doses of corticosteroids may be required.

Disease course
- May require treatment for many years.
- 50% recovered at 3 years.
- Durations of 15 years are reported.
- 5–25% will develop giant cell arteritis which practically never supervenes in PMR once patient is under adequate corticosteroid treatment.

Giant cell (temporal) arteritis (GCA)
As sudden and irreversible blindness may occur, treatment should be commenced immediately.

Pathology
Pan-arteritis, often segmental, consisting of:
- Necrosis of artery wall.
- Fragmentation of internal elastic lamina.
- Granulomata containing giant cells.

Clinical features (Table 5.8)
- Elderly >70 years.
- Polymyalgia rheumatica as prodrome in 40%.
- Loss of weight.
- Headache, commonly unilateral.
- Scalp tenderness; painful to brush the hair or wear a hat.
- Temporal arteries may show tender beaded thickening and/or loss of pulsation.

5 Important rheumatological conditions

5.6 Polymyalgia rheumatica and giant cell arteritis

Table 5.8 Clinical features of giant cell arteritis

Clinical feature	%	Clinical feature	%
Headache	70	Anaemia	20
Weight loss	50	Swollen scalp arteries	20
Loss of temporal artery pulsation	45	Arterial bruits	20
		Visual loss	15
Jaw claudication	45	Synovitis	15
Fatigue	40	CNS abnormalities	15
Fever	40	Carotid sinus sensitivity	10
PMR	40	Swallowing claudication	10
Artery tenderness	30	Tongue claudication	5
Visual symptoms	30		

- Disturbance of vision.
- Jaw claudication.
- Arterial bruits particularly in neck, axillae and femoral canal regions.

Investigations

1 ESR almost invariably raised >100 mm/h.
2 Temporal artery biopsy:
   histological changes patchy;
   25% have normal histology despite bilateral biopsy and multiple sections;
   if it is performed should be done early as corticosteroids will reverse changes.
3 Anticardiolipin antibodies in 60%.

Management

1 Treatment should be instituted immediately.
2 40 mg prednisolone EC daily.
3 Biopsy confirmation may be obtained later if required.
4 Follow-up according to patient's symptoms and ESR, the dose of prednisolone may be reduced in 5 mg steps to 15 mg and then by 1 mg steps.

5 Important rheumatological conditions

5.6 Polymyalgia rheumatica and giant cell arteritis

Disease course
As long as myalgic and arteritic symptoms are controlled, serious complications are avoided even if the ESR is not completely normal.

Atypical presentations of GCA
1 Stroke: high ESR indicates that atherosclerosis is not the underlying pathology.
2 Pulseless disease or aortic arch syndromes (polymyalgia arteritica).
3 15% may present with PUO, marked weight loss and be extensively investigated for malignancy ('masked GCA'). Temporal artery biopsy may make diagnosis.

5 Important rheumatological conditions

5.7 Bone disease

5.7 Bone disease

Osteoporosis

Definition
Reduction of total bone mass below that expected for age and sex.

Prevalence
Osteoporosis is common especially in the elderly female population. The clinical presentations of fracture of the proximal femur and vertebral crush fractures contribute to morbidity and death in this age group.

Aetiology
Total bone mass rises to a maximum during the third decade and is positively influenced by adequate exercise and calcium intake. From age 35 there is then a slow decline in bone mass plus in women there is a rapid loss associated with the menopause. Table 5.9 shows factors influencing the development of osteoporosis.

Clinical features
Related to presence of complications or underlying disease.
1 Habitus: protruberant abdomen, thoracic kyphosis which if severe may cause respiratory embarrassment. Pain may result from impingement of lower ribs on the iliac crest.
2 Recurrent fractures; hip, wrist and vertebral are the more frequent.
3 Pain from vertebral crush fractures:
   usually acute, resolving over 2–6 weeks;
   spreads around body from back to anterior chest and abdomen;
   walking and sitting up difficult;
   tenderness to light percussion over affected vertebra;

5 Important rheumatological conditions

5.7 Bone disease

Table 5.9. Causes of osteoporosis

> 1 Juvenile osteoporosis
> 2 Idiopathic senile osteoporosis
> 3 Postmenopausal osteoporosis
> 4 Chronic liver disease
> 5 Chronic inflammatory and disabling disease Rheumatoid arthritis, multiple sclerosis
> 6 Endocrine disorders
>   Hyperparathyroidism
>   Hyperthyroidism
>   Cushing's syndrome
>   Hypogonadism
>   Hypopituitarism
>   Chronic diabetes mellitus
> 7 Drugs
>   Corticosteroids
>   Alcohol
>   Smoking
> 8 Multiple myeloma
> 9 Local osteoporosis
>   Disuse and paralysis
>   Sudek's atrophy
>   Regional migratory osteoporosis

resulting postural problems may lead to chronic pain.
4 Loss of height.

Investigations

Laboratory tests are normal in osteoporosis and are performed to exclude other causes of bone pain or predisposing factors.

X-rays (Figs 5.15, 5.16):

1 Osteoporosis; 30% of bone mass lost before loss of density shows on radiographs.
2 For fractures.

Dual photon densitometry dual energy X-ray or computerized X-ray tomography is carried out for bone mass.

5 Important rheumatological conditions

5.7 Bone disease

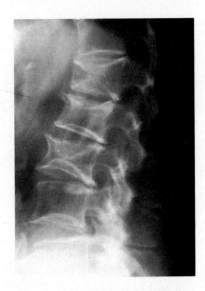

Fig. 5.15 Marked senile osteoporosis showing multiple end-plate compression fractures giving 'codfish' vertebrae, thin cortex and simplified trabecular pattern.

Bone biopsy will confirm the presence of osteoporosis and exclude concurrent osteomalacia. The rate of mineralization of bone is demonstrated by tetracycline labelling (see section 7.2).

Management
Prevention is all important.
1 Adequate calcium intake; recommended daily allowance 800 mg daily, 1500 mg in middle aged females.
2 Adequate exercise especially in period of growth.
3 Hormone replacement therapy (HRT) using oestrogen/progestrogen in cyclical fashion should be given to women with early menopause. This is the only clearly proven preventative treatment for loss of bone mass and of fractures.
4 Vitamin supplements. It seems reasonable that patients with

5 Important rheumatological conditions

5.7 Bone disease

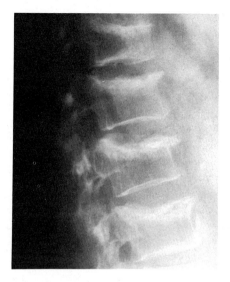

Fig. 5.16 Steroid associated osteoporosis of the spine showing multiple end-plate fractures within adjacent abundant callus formation, vertebral wedging and osteopenia.

RA and on corticosteroids should receive calcium supplements and a small amount of vitamin D: calcium gluconate 4.5 g t.d.s. (400 mg calcium); calcium and vitamin D BP one tablet daily.
5 Calcitonin has been granted a licence in the USA and has shown benefit in short-term use. It is safe but expensive.
6 There is now evidence that sodium fluoride 20–25 mg/day is helpful. It should be given together with calcium and vitamin D.
7 Anabolic steroids and bisphosphonates are experimental but promising.

Osteomalacia
This is important as it may cause non-specific aches and pains, but will respond to treatment.

5 Important rheumatological conditions

5.7 Bone disease

Definition
Histological appearance of widened osteoid seams on undecalcified sections of bone.

Aetiology
Due to lack of 1,25 vitamin D.
1 Nutritional causes:
  inadequate dietary intake;
  lack of exposure to sunshine;
  total or partial gastrectomy;
  jejunal malabsorption;
    pancreatic disease;
    coeliac disease;
    tropical sprue;
    blind loop syndrome;
    systemic sclerosis.
2 Renal disease:
  Fanconi's syndrome;
  renal tubular acidosis;
  Wilson's disease;
  chronic pyelonephritis.

Clinical features
1 High risk groups: the very elderly and coloured immigrants.
2 Poorly localized pain:
  characteristically affects shoulders, low back and thighs;
  painful limitation of movement on weight-bearing contrasts with free movement when the same limbs are examined with the patient supine on the couch.
3 Weakness of proximal muscles.
4 Dorsal kyphosis.
5 In childhood (rickets):
  growth retardation;
  enlargement of cartilagenous epiphyses which fail to ossify;
  curved bones;

5 Important rheumatological conditions

5.7 Bone disease

varus or valgus knees;
prominent foreheads;
enlarged costal cartilages, 'rickety rosary';
scoliosis.

Differential diagnosis
1 Polymyalgia rheumatica.
2 OA hips.
3 Paget's disease of the pelvis.
4 Disseminated bone metastases.

Investigations
1 *Dietary assessment.*
2 *Laboratory:*
   (a) FBC and plasma viscosity;
   (b) urea and electrolytes;
   (c) serum calcium studies; low calcium, low phosphate, raised alkaline phosphatase;
   (d) red cell folate;
   (e) β-carotenoids.
3 *X-rays* (Fig. 5.17):
   (a) pseudofractures or Looser's zones seen (the adult presentation of hypophosphatasia may show similar radiographic appearances; it is distinguished biochemically by a normal serum calcium and phosphate, low alkaline phosphatase and raised phosphoethanolamine in the urine);
       ischial and pubic rami;
       through ilium;
       lateral edge of scapula;
       neck and shaft of tibia, fibula and metatarsals;
   (b) spine 'codfish' vertebrae.
4 *Bone biopsy* preceded by tetracycline labelling shows widening of the osteoid seams.

5 Important rheumatological conditions

5.7 Bone disease

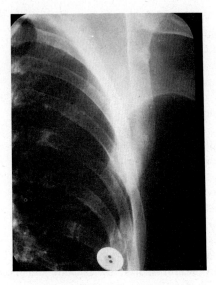

Fig. 5.17 Osteomalacia in a 35-year-old male with Crohn's disease showing pseudo fractures (Looser's zones) affecting left scapula and ribs, and osteopenia.

Management
1 Dihydrotachysterol (Tachyrol) 2 mg per day.
2 Alphacalcidol (1-alpha) 1 µg per day (for those with renal disease).

There are three outcome measures for the results of treatment:
1 Cessation of bone pain on weight bearing usually occurs within 2 weeks.
2 Normalization of serum calcium.
3 Normalization of alkaline phosphatase.

Note that there is a danger of overdosage from vitamin D derivatives. The serum alkaline phosphatase is the best indicator of adequate treatment. It falls towards normal before the serum calcium rises to a toxic level. At that point the dose is reduced to

5 Important rheumatological conditions

5.7 Bone disease

2 mg dihydrotachysterol weekly for maintenance. Monthly or 2-monthly checks of calcium and alkaline phosphatase are then required.

Hyperparathyroidism

Aetiology
1 Over-secretion of parathyroid hormone (parathormone, PTH), secondary to:
   parathyroid gland hypertrophy;
   parathyroid tumours, benign or (rarely) malignant;
   part of a pturiglandular syndrome, with other secretary tumours in adrenal, pancreas, thyroid and elsewhere;
   chronic renal disease.
leading to:
   raised circulating levels of PTH;
   hypernatraemia and hypercalciuria;
   hyperphosphaturia.
2 Most common in older females.

Clinical features
1 Those caused by hypercalcaemia:
   polyuria — may resemble diabetes insipidis;
   nephrocalcinosis;
   kidney stones;
   chondrocalcinosis (pseudogout);
   muscular weakness;
   mental disturbances; varying from lethargy through psychoses to coma.
2 Those caused by associated renal failure:
   Raised blood urea, creatinine, urate. Urate gout, tendency to infective pyelitis.
3 Those caused by increased bone resorption to compensate for urinary calcium loss:
   radiological osteoporosis;

5 Important rheumatological conditions

5.7 Bone disease

fibrocystic disease of bone;
subperiosteal erosion of bone in fingers (see Fig. 5.18), ends of clavicles and elsewhere;
loss of lamina dura in dental X-ray.

4 Mild hyperparathyroidism may be asymptomatic — picked up on routine serum calcium measurements.

5 Rarely, a parathyroid tumour is palpable in the neck or seen on lateral soft tissue X-ray of the neck.

6 Pain — various causes: bones and joints may ache and be stiff. Arthritis with swelling of joints is due to crystal arthropathy from calcium pyrophosphate dihydrate, urate or mixed crystals.

7 Gastrointestinal symptoms include nausea, vomiting, constipation and anorexia.

8 Associated conditions include gastric and duodenal ulceration and pancreatitis.

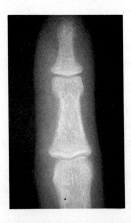

Fig. 5.18 Hyperparathyroidism showing subperiostial erosion affecting the proximal phalanx, loss of cortico-medullary junction, and lacey trabecular pattern.

5 Important rheumatological conditions

5.7 Bone disease

Investigations
1 Blood:
   serum immunoreactive PTH;
   serum calcium;
   alkaline phosphatase;
   urea, creatinine, uric acid.
2 Urine:
   calcium:creatinine ratio;
   phosphate:creatinine ratio;
   uralysis.
3 X-ray (see Fig. 5.18):
   skeletal screen;
   hands for subperiostial erosions;
   abdomen on CT scan for nephrocalcinosis;
   jaws for loss of lamina dura.

Management
1 Exclude other causes of hypercalcaemia such as malignancy (especially myeloma, hypernephroma and breast cancer) or vitamin D intoxication.
2 Mild disease (asymptomatic, serum Ca < 3 mmol/l) — observation only.
3 More severe disease — surgery.

Osteonecrosis

Aetiology
This condition results from death of bone cells due to loss of blood supply or ionizing radiation. Increased intra-osseous pressure appears to be an important mechanism. The subchondral bone of the joints is the most vulnerable to osteonecrosis. The aetiology includes the following.
1 Avascular necrosis (post-trauma).
2 Idiopathic osteonecrosis.
3 Excess glucocorticoids.

5 Important rheumatological conditions

5.7 Bone disease

4 SLE.
5 Haemoglobinopathies.
6 Metabolic disease:
   diabetes;
   haemochromatosis;
   Gaucher's disease;
   alcoholism;
   pancreatitis;
   fat embolism;
   hyperlipidaemia;
   hyperviscosity;
   bismuth intoxication.
7 Radiotherapy.
8 Caisson disease (barotrauma).

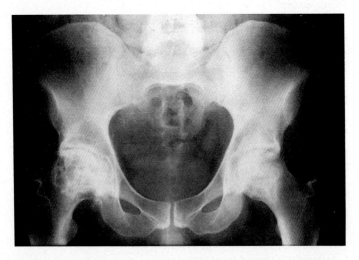

Fig. 5.19 Osteo-avascular necrosis — radiograph showing extensive zones of radiolucency with marginal sclerosis throughout the femoral head and neck, and secondary OA on right.

5 Important rheumatological conditions

5.7 Bone disease

Clinical features
1 Sites involved:
  femoral head;
  humeral head;
  femoral condyles;
  tibial plateau;
  talus;
  scaphoid (post-trauma) and lunate;
  metatarsal and metacarpal heads (SLE).
2 Pain in affected part, although early stages asymptomatic.
3 Secondary osteoarthritis.

Investigations
1 X-rays (Fig. 5.19):

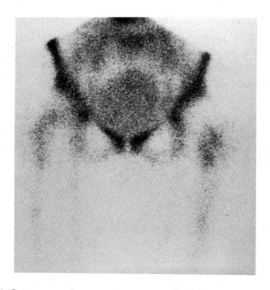

Fig. 5.20 Osteo-avascular necrosis — nanocolloid bone scan showing marked deficiency of activity in L femoral head and neck.

181

5 Important rheumatological conditions

5.7 Bone disease

stage I, absent changes apart from occasional osteoporosis;
stage II, sclerotic zone adjacent to lucent region in subchondral bone — the 'crescent sign';
stage III, irregular bone density with collapse of articular surface;
stage IV, joint destruction and osteoarthritic change.
2 Radioisotope bone scanning detects abnormalities before there is radiographic change (Fig. 5.20).
3 MRI (see Fig. 3.1, p. 64) detects the earliest bony changes.

Management

1 Medical: Analgesia and NSAIDs together with 6 months non weight bearing and 6 months partial weight bearing (hip). Unsatisfactory once radiographic changes have occurred.
2 Surgical:
   (a) decompression by removal of core of cancellous bone followed by protective weight bearing for 6 weeks, increased for 4 to 6 weeks, then unrestricted;
   (b) bone grafting;
   (c) osteotomy;
   (d) joint replacement.

Note that disease is *bilateral* in 66% with idiopathic disease of the femoral head. Earliest treatment means the best outcome, so the other hip must be watched carefully in a patient with unilateral hip disease.

Paget's disease

Definition
A unifocal or multifocal disorder of bone with irregular osteoporosis accompanied by new bone formation.

5 Important rheumatological conditions

5.7 Bone disease

Aetiology
Unknown. Measles-like viral particles are observed in affected bone. There is a striking geographical distribution. It is common in Britain (5% of skeletons in Lancashire) but very rare in China.

Clinical features
1 Elderly mainly affected.
2 Often asymptomatic — chance radiographic finding.
3 Bone pain is often nocturnal and not positional.
4 Skeletal abnormalities:
   bowing of the tibia;
   skull enlargement;
   spinal involvement with loss of height (kyphosis or scoliosis) and spinal stenosis;
   affected bones may be warm from increased blood flow.
5 Nerve compression syndromes.
6 Joint incongruity may lead to osteoarthritis.
7 Pathological fractures common.
8 Deafness (due to otosclerosis).
9 High output cardiac failure.
10 Bone sarcoma may supervene in 1%.

Investigations
1 Alkaline phosphatase (bone origin) can be very high.
2 Increased urinary hydroxyproline excretion (normal = 22–77 mg/24 h).
3 X-rays characteristic: films of pelvis, upper femur and skull are best for screening (Fig. 5.21).

Treatment
1 Symptomatic — analgesics if mild disease.
2 Calcitonin — if severe administer a dose range of 80 IU 3 times weekly to 160 IU daily. Side effects include nausea, vomiting and

5 Important rheumatological conditions

5.7 Bone disease

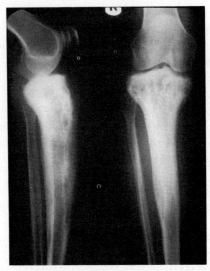

Fig. 5.21 Paget's disease involving the right tibia showing patchy sclerosis with bony expansion and anterior bowing, loss of cortico-medullary differentiation and V-shaped resorption front.

facial flushing which may be reduced with pizotifen. Monitor clinical improvement which usually occurs within 3 months but may be delayed, and biochemistry — urinary hydroxyproline falls within days, alkaline phosphatase within weeks.

3 Etidronate disodium:
   dose 5 mg/kg for not longer than 6 months;
   take at least 2 h away from food;
   side-effects: high doses can cause osteomalacia;
   avoid in renal impairment and in colitis.

Algodystrophy (Sudeck's atrophy)

Aetiology
1 Idiopathic in 50%.
2 Trauma.

3 Nerve root or peripheral nerve lesions.
4 Ischaemic heart disease.

Clinical features
1 Uncommon.
2 Equal sex incidence, any age.
3 Acute phase — burning pain, swelling and loss of function of affected region, usually hand or foot. Vasomotor changes cause coldness (rarely warm flushing). Stiffness of the ipsilateral shoulder may accompany hand disease (shoulder–hand syndrome).
4 Dystrophic phase — resolution of pain and swelling after weeks or months leaving trophic skin changes.
5 Atrophic phase — subcutaneous atrophy and flexion contractures may occur 3–6 months later.

Investigations
1 Laboratory investigations normal.
2 X-rays: regional osteoporosis develops after a few weeks.
3 Radioisotope bone scan shows increased uptake before X-ray changes.

Management
1 Physiotherapy — vigorous mobilization therapy essential in the acute phase.
2 Corticosteroids — a short course may be helpful.
3 Sympathetic blockade using guanethidine may relieve pain and swelling.

Disease course
There is a variable course and early treatment may reduce risk of subsequent atrophy. Recovery in 1–2 years in 75%.

5 Important rheumatological conditions

5.8 Infective arthritis

The normal joint is remarkably resistant to infection. Infection may cause arthritis in four ways:
1 Blood-borne infection.
2 Contaminated direct penetration by a thorn, needle aspiration, surgery.
3 Local extension (rare) from osteomyelitis.
4 Reactive arthritis (see section 5.3).

Acute pyogenic arthritis
This is a medical emergency which untreated may be life-threatening; delayed treatment can lead to severe joint destruction. Onset may be insidious and atypical. It may be mistaken for a localized flare-up of pre-existing chronic arthritis, particularly in chronic rheumatoid arthritis.

Aetiology
- Most pyogenic infection is due to *Staphylococcus aureus*. Others include:
  Streptococcus pyogenes;
  Staphylococcus albus;
  Haemophilus influenzae;
  Pseudomonas aeruginosa;
  Escherichia coli.
- Systemic predisposing factors include:
  diabetes;
  rheumatoid arthritis;
  leukaemia;
  myelomatosis;
  immunosuppressive treatment;
  corticosteroid therapy;
  intravenous drug abuse;
  acquired immune deficiency syndrome (AIDS).
- Local factors include:
  joint aspiration;

5 Important rheumatological conditions

5.8 Infective arthritis

surgery;
joint damage from arthritis.

Clinical features
- Acute onset in 25%.
- Subacute in remainder and patient may be non-toxic.
- More common in very young and elderly.
- Hip and knee most common joints.
- Others include wrist, shoulder, ankle, wrist.
- Pain in region of involved joint.
- Exacerbated by movement.
- Heat and swelling of one or more joints.
- Patient generally ill.
- Pyrexia.
- Spasm in muscles controlling joint.
- Marked tenderness.
- Effusion.
- Thirty per cent have > 1 joint involved.
- Spinal disease is occult.
- Pain may be the sole sign of hip involvement.

Investigations
1 *Joint aspiration.* Send immediately for microscopy and Gram stain, culture and sensitivity. Inject portion into blood culture bottles. Synovial white count is usually high (> 50 000/mm^3); synovial fluid lactate is raised but has poor specificity. Note that the presence of crystals (urate, pyrophosphate) does not exclude infection as the cause of joint inflammation.
2 *Blood cultures.* Swab any possible source of infection.
3 *FBC* and viscosity: these can be normal, and do not exclude a septic joint.
4 *X-ray* changes late: 1–2 weeks (see Fig. 5.22):
osteoporosis;
joint space narrowing;
subluxation;

5 Important rheumatological conditions

5.8 Infective arthritis

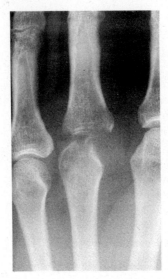

Fig. 5.22 Septic arthritis affecting a MCP joint showing ill-defined soft tissue swelling, marked juxta-articular osteoporosis, and bone destruction both sides of the joint margin.

erosion of articular cortices.
5 *Bone scintigraphy*: will detect changes before X-rays and is helpful for axial joints including spine and hip.

Management
A good outcome requires prompt diagnosis and treatment. A high index of suspicion is needed especially in high-risk groups who can present atypically.
1 *Systemic antibiotics*. Give immediately according to Gram stain result. Modify once the nature and sensitivity of the organism is known (Table 5.10). They should be administered intravenously for at least 2 weeks and then orally for a further 2−4 weeks.
2 *Aspiration of joint*. The joint should be aspirated regularly. This

5 Important rheumatological conditions

5.8 Infective arthritis

removes bacterial debris and relieves pain through the reduction of intra-articular pressures.

3 *Surgical drainage* if:
pus cannot be aspirated completely;
inaccessible joint, especially the hip;
failure of medical treatment.

4 *Rest* the involved joint in a plaster shell leaving access for aspiration.

5 *Physiotherapy*: passive and non-weight-bearing, then active as pain subsides.

Complications
1 Bone involvement.
2 Recurrent infection.
3 Bony ankylosis.
4 Limb length inequality (children).
5 Destructive arthritis.

Table 5.10. Suggested antibiotic regimes (modified from Dieppe *et al.* 1985)

Result of Gram stain	Suggested systemic antibiotic and dosage	
Gram-positive cocci	Flucloxacillin	0.5–1 g q.d.s.
	Cefuroxime	2 g q.d.s.
Gram-negative cocci	Ampicillin	0.5 g q.d.s.
Gram-negative bacilli	Gentamicin	80 mg q.d.s. (levels required)
	Carbenicillin	5 g q.d.s.
Unknown	Flucloxacillin and gentamicin	

Note: drugs and dosages are intended as a guide only
Consult with microbiologist and pharmacist
Dosage modified in the very young, elderly and those with renal impairment

5 Important rheumatological conditions

5.8 Infective arthritis

Infection in a prosthetic joint
The enormous success of hip replacement and to a lesser extent other joint replacements has brought its own problems.

Frequency (0.5–2%) of infected hip prostheses:

40% present early	(0–2 months)
45% are delayed	(2–24 months)
15% are late	(> 24 months)

Aetiology
Organisms include:

Staphylococcus aureus }
Staphylococcus albus } 66%
Streptococcus 20%;
Gram-negative 10%;
others — anaerobes, mixed, unusual, e.g. *Listeria monocytogenes*.

Clinical features
1 The presentation is often subacute and may occur months or even years after operation.
2 Pain with or without swelling in affected joint.
3 Fever.
4 Slight warmth and boggy swelling may persist for several months following joint replacement without indicating infection.

Investigations
1 Examination of synovial fluid (as above). Inform the surgeon, aspirate the joint using strict aseptic techniques. The organism may not be isolated.
2 Laboratory:
FBC — only 10% have a raised WCC;
ESR not specific, may be normal;
blood cultures;
swab possible source sites.

5 Important rheumatological conditions

5.8 Infective arthritis

3 X-rays.
4 Bone scanning using gallium and technetium.
5 Surgery — the main differential diagnosis is between pain due to sepsis or due to loosening. On occasions, the definitive diagnosis is only made at operation.

Management
1 Prophylactic administration of antibiotics during dental and other procedures.
2 Prolonged antibiotic treatment required.
3 May require removal of prosthesis.

Septic arthritis due to specific causes

Gonococcal arthritis
This is the commonest form of infective arthritis in many countries especially the USA.

Clinical features
Predominantly female (F:M = 4:1).
1 Joints:
   tenosynovitis;
   initially abrupt onset, polyarthritis;
   asymmetrical, migratory then may settle as established mono-oligoarticular arthritis;
   effusions common.
2 Skin:
   rash (70%) papules becoming vesiculopustular;
   tender, mainly limbs.
3 Fever.
4 Pericarditis, meningitis and osteomyelitis may occur.

Investigations
Neisseria gonorrhoea is extremely fastidious and care must be taken in attempting to isolate the organism. Appropriate

5 Important rheumatological conditions

5.8 Infective arthritis

specimens should be taken immediately to the laboratory.
1 Swabs: cervical, urethral, rectal and pharyngeal plated onto Theyer—Martin plates (selective medium).
2 Aspiration of synovial fluid: plate on to chocolate agar; are positive in 50%.
3 Blood cultures — plate sample on to chocolate agar; remainder in culture bottles.
4 Gonoccocal fixation tests cannot distinguish recent from distant infection.

Management
1 Antibiotics: Penicillin G 2.5 megaunits q.d.s. until asymptomatic, then ampicillin 500 mg q.d.s. orally for 10 days (use cefuroxime, or spectinomycin if penicillin-allergic).
2 Contact tracing.

The organism causing infective arthritis is very sensitive to penicillin. A few case reports now exist of resistant organisms which can be treated with spectinomycin.

Meningococcal arthritis
Sporadic and epidemic outbreaks. Children are affected more often than adults.

Clinical features
Three forms exist.
1 Direct infection of joints causing destructive arthritis. Usually part of life-threatening acute meningococcal septicaemia (fever, meningitis, purpuric rash, adrenal failure, toxic shock).
2 Subacute reactive arthritis (joint fluid culture negative) with no residual joint damage (usually part of chronic meningococcal septicaemia).
3 Arthralgias associated with fever without joint swelling.

Investigations
Culture CSF, throat swabs, blood and joint fluid.

5 Important rheumatological conditions

5.8 Infective arthritis

Management
- Intravenous benzylpenicillin 20/30 mg/kg body weight 4-hourly for 7 days, or chloramphenicol in penicillin-sensitive patients.
- Treatment of acute forms is urgent — treat on clinical diagnosis. Don't wait for results of cultures.
- Give intra-articular antibiotics only if joint fluid culture is positive.
- Chemoprophylaxis of contacts as advised by microbiologist.

Mycobacterium tuberculosis
Worldwide one of the commonest causes of infective arthritis.

Clinical features
- Insidious onset.
- Gradual increase of pain and swelling.
- Usually monoarticular.
- Hip and knee most common peripheral joints.
- Spine occasionally involved.
- More common in immigrants and elderly.

Investigations
- Synovial fluid culture.
- Synovial biopsy for culture and histology.
- Sputum culture.
- Three early morning urine samples.
- X-rays: CXR, joint (see Fig. 5.23).

Management
1 Antibiotics: combination anti-tuberculous chemotherapy, continue with two agents for 18 months.
2 Surgical synovectomy and drainage in later disease.

Lyme disease
First recognized in 1975 in Old Lyme, Connecticut, USA. Cases are now reported in Europe and UK.

Infection usually occurs in summer with a rash, erythema

5 Important rheumatological conditions

5.8 Infective arthritis

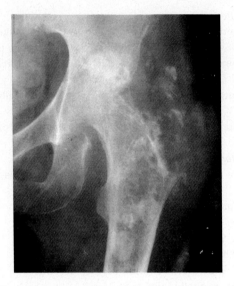

Fig. 5.23 TB arising in the trochanteric bursa and spreading to the hip showing amorphous soft tissue calcification, 'cold abscess' and total ablation of the articular surfaces.

chronicum migrans, which may be followed by neurological, cardiac or articular complications.

Persistent and severe disease is associated with HLA DR2.

Aetiology
The disease is caused by *Borellia burgdorferi* carried by ticks (*Ixodes dammini* in USA).

Clinical features
1 Equal sex incidence, median age 28 years.
2 Skin. Erythema chronicum migrans starts as papular or macular lesion, at tick bite, and enlarges to become annular with

5 Important rheumatological conditions

5.8 Infective arthritis

an outer red margin and central induration. Thigh, groin and axilla are common initial sites. There are multiple lesions in 50% and the rash fades within 3–4 weeks, but can recur. Rash is accompanied by fever, myalgia, lymphadenopathy and malaise.
3 Joint pains (60%) occur from a few weeks to 2 years after bite. There is early migratory arthropathy and later recurrent oligoarthropathy with effusions usually affecting the knee and other large joints.

Complications
1 Neurological (15%). The most common is a fluctuating meningoencephalitis with cranial and peripheral neuropathies which may last for several months and be recurrent, although there is complete resolution.
2 Cardiac (8%):
   fluctuating AV block;
   myo-and pericarditis may occur;
   short duration, may recur.

Investigations
1 Raised ESR.
2 Mild anaemia and leucocytosis.
3 Raised LDH and SGOT.
4 Microscopic haematuria and proteinuria.
5 Renal function tests normal.
6 Organism may be recovered from blood, skin and CSF.
7 Serum IgM antibody rises in 3–6 weeks.
8 IgG peaks several months after infection.

Treatment
Symptomatic treatment for complications. Initial infection treated with tetracycline, 250–500 mg q.d.s.

5 Important rheumatological conditions

5.8 Infective arthritis

Fungal infections of joints

Various fungal infections have been described as causing arthritis. These include:
- aspergillosis;
- blastomycosis;
- candidiasis;
- coccidiomycosis;
- cryptococcosis;
- histoplasmosis;
- mycetoma pedis infection (Madura foot);
- sporotrichosis.

Joint involvement usually occurs as part of a generalized fungal infection, often in immunocompromised hosts. Biopsy and culture of synovium is required for diagnosis.

Management
This involves treatment with appropriate antifungal agents.

Viral arthritis

Various viruses are associated with arthritis (Table 5.11). The arthritis is usually of acute onset, polyarticular, and self-limiting with no joint destruction. However, occasionally symptoms may persist and cause diagnostic confusion. Diagnosis depends on serological testing and treatment is symptomatic.

AIDS and arthritis

A painful arthritis, seronegative for rheumatoid factor may occur early in AIDS and may be the presenting symptom. Knees most often affected. Pain relief with intra-articular corticosteroids. Later a wide variety of secondary bacterial, fungal or viral infections causing arthritis may occur.

5 Important rheumatological conditions

5.8 Infective arthritis

Table 5.11. Features of viral arthritis

Virus	Clinical features	Natural history
Rubella	Rapid onset, polyarticular. Occurs before and after rash and may also follow vaccination	Joint symptoms last 3–14 days, can last up to 1 year
Mumps	Males most often affected, migratory, usually large joints	Clears within 10 days
Parvovirus	Females, acute polyarthritis with rash and flu-like symptoms. IgM antibody raised for 3 months	Usually self-limiting, can be recurrent
Hepatitis B	Occur as prodrome in 10–25% of hepatitis B infection. Abrupt onset, polyarticular, fever and vasculitic skin rash	Joint symptoms resolve after 3 weeks often at onset of jaundice, may be recurrent in persistent antigenaemia

5 Important rheumatological conditions

5.9 Trauma and haemorrhage

Bone fractures

It is not uncommon for elderly arthritics to present to doctors with pain arising near a joint which is easily misdiagnosed as an exacerbation of arthritis, but is in reality a fracture. March fractures (metatarsals) and scaphoid (carpal) fractures are particularly likely to be misdiagnosed.

Aetiology

Risk factors include:
1 Osteoporosis and/or osteomalacia.
2 Difficulty in walking due to joint disease.
3 Poor eyesight and balance.
4 Confusion.
5 Drugs, especially corticosteroids.
6 Paget's disease.
7 Bony metastases.

Clinical features

Table 5.12 shows common sites for fractures.
- Pain, swelling.
- Bone instability: impaction of the fracture may mask this sign.
- Stress fractures may be detected by pencil rolling test (see section 1.2).

Investigations

1 FBC viscosity.
2 Urea and electrolytes.
3 Liver function tests.
4 Calcium studies.
5 X-rays.

Management

See Table 5.12.

5 Important rheumatological conditions

5.9 Trauma and haemorrhage

Table 5.12. Common fractures and their management

Fracture	Management
Colles' and Burnett's fractures	Reduction and immobilization in extension
Impacted fractures of proximal radius and humerus	Use of a sling
Proximal femur	Pinning or joint replacement
Tibial plateau crush fractures	Joint replacement or osteotomy
Stress fractures of ankle and feet	Period of non weight bearing

Despite underlying bone disease, fractures heal in usual time with standard treatment

Haemorrhage into joints

Haemarthrosis implies trauma, but in rheumatology this is often trauma on top of pre-existing inflammatory arthritis, osteoarthritis or chondrocalcinosis.

Haemarthrosis of the knee

Aetiology
1 Trauma:
  road traffic accidents;
  skiing injury;
2 Bleeding disorders — haemophilia.
3 Intra and juxta-articular tumours:
  haemangioma;
  villonodular synovitis;
  synovioma;
  osteosarcoma.
4 Joint disease:
  rheumatoid arthritis;

5 Important rheumatological conditions

5.9 Trauma and haemorrhage

chondrocalcinosis;
osteoarthritis.

Clinical features
1 Pain and rapid swelling of knee.
2 Restriction of movement.

Investigations
1 FBC and viscosity.
2 Clotting studies.
3 Microscopy and culture of synovial fluid.
4 Cytology if appropriate.
5 X-ray.

Management

Trauma. Aspirate sufficient blood to decompress the joint. Use ice packs to stop the bleeding and immobilize knee in a padded plaster at 5° flexion.

Seek surgical advice with transverse and stellate fracture of the patella or when there is evidence of cruciate or collateral ligamentous rupture.

Haemophilia. Apply ice packs to affected joint, give Factor VIII and aspirate blood from joint once bleeding tendency has been corrected.

Note that frequently the most painful joints contain relatively little blood as the haemorrhage has been into bone rather than the joint cavity.

Knee contractures may be straightened by manipulation or serial splinting.

5   Important rheumatological conditions

5.10 Paediatric rheumatology

5.10 Paediatric rheumatology

Children may commonly complain of joint pains, although arthritis is rare. When arthritis does occur it is generally short-lived and resolves spontaneously.

Non-arthritic causes of musculoskeletal pain include 'growing pains', which are recurrent limb pains typically waking the child at night. Examination is normal and there is generally an underlying emotional disturbance.

Other causes of joint pains include non-accidental injury and hypermobility.

Chronic arthritis
Arthritis lasting longer than 3 months, which ccours in 1/1000 children.

Juvenile chronic arthritis (JCA)
Also called: Still's disease, juvenile rheumatoid arthritis (USA).

The classification is based on the mode of onset of disease.

systemic	20%
polyarticular (≥4 joints)	15%
pauciarticular (<4 joints)	65%

Systemic onset

Clinical features

1 Sex incidence equal; age of onset 1–4, rare after 6 years.
2 Fever: remittent, high during the evening, often normal during the day. Persists more than 3 weeks.
3 Rash: transient, maculo-papular, occurs with fever.
4 Lymphadenopathy common, especially epitrochlear, axillary and mesentric nodes (may cause abdominal pain).
5 Splenomegaly (50%), hepatomegaly (10%).
6 Pericarditis.
7 Joint symptoms may be absent initially, but 50% will develop polyarthritis especially involving knees, wrists and ankles.

5 Important rheumatological conditions

5.10 Paediatric rheumatology

Differential diagnosis
1 Infections.
2 Occult malignancy.
3 Rheumatic fever.
4 Connective tissue diseases.

Investigations
- Clinical diagnosis, no diagnostic test.
- Raised ESR (> 100 mm/h).
- High WCC, platelets.

Course and prognosis
- Fifty per cent resolve after 3 months.
- Remainder develop polyarthritis.
- Mortality 7% from intercurrent infection or amyloidosis.

Polyarticular onset

Clinical features
1 Predominantly females; age 8–10 years.
2 Joints: onset acute or subacute:
   symmetrical polyarthritis affecting hands, knees, wrists and ankles;
   neck and temporo-mandibular joint involvement also seen;
   occasionally contractures may occur without overt synovitis.
3 Systemic features minimal or absent.

Differential diagnosis
1 Psoriatic arthritis.
2 Connective tissue diseases.
3 Haemoglobinopathies.
4 Sarcoidosis.
5 Reactive arthritis.

5 Important rheumatological conditions

5.10 Paediatric rheumatology

Investigations
1 ESR and CRP raised.
2 X-ray: changes late as thicker cartilage is found in childhood. Erosions are rare. There is growth retardation with chronic disease — this affects the whole skeleton. Local growth changes — growth is sometimes accelerated by epiphyseal hyperaemia near affected joints. Later, premature ossification of epiphyses causes local growth failure.

Course and prognosis
Subacute onset and early disease has a poor prognosis. Arthritis settles in teenage with good functional outcome.

Pauciarticular onset

Clinical features
1 Predominantly females; age under 5 years.
2 Joints involved: knee, ankle, elbow, neck and wrist; monoarthritis involving finger or toe may occur.
3 Eyes: posterior uveitis, bilateral in 2/3, associated with ANA. Often asymptomatic until blindness (60% untreated).

Differential diagnosis
1 Septic arthritis.
2 Arthritis of inflammatory bowel disease.
3 Hypogammaglobulinaemia.
4 Pigmented villonodular synovitis.
5 Plant thorn synovitis.

Investigations
1 ESR normal or slightly raised.
2 ANA 30%.
3 X-rays normal initially; later, asymmetric growth defects may be evident.

5 Important rheumatological conditions

5.10 Paediatric rheumatology

Course and prognosis
Thirty-five per cent of patients are in remission at 5 years. There is seldom severe functional limitation in the remainder.

Juvenile ankylosing spondylitis

Ten per cent of adult AS is of juvenile onset and there is a family history in 75%.

Clinical features
1 M:F = 5:1; age of onset >9 years.
2 Joints: no back pain initially; presents with pauciarticular pattern (hips, knee, ankle and toes); achilles tendinitis, plantar fasciitis and occasionally neck stiffness may be sole manifestations of joint disease.
3 Eyes: iridocyclitis 25%.
4 Other: aortic incompetence, bowel disease and psoriasis are rare.

Investigations
1 HLA B27 (90%).
2 X-rays: appearance of sacroiliitis delayed for several years.

Course and prognosis
There is generally a good prognosis. Hip involvement determines functional outcome, although limitation of spinal movement, toe deformities and restricted subtalar movement may occur.

Juvenile rheumatoid arthritis

Clinical features
1 Females predominate; age of onset >10 years.
2 Joints: symmetrical polyarthritis. The distribution is as in adult RA and early deformities are common. Hip involvement is more frequent than in adults and nodules and other extra-articular manifestations are common.

5 Important rheumatological conditions

5.10 Paediatric rheumatology

Investigations
1 ESR and CRP raised.
2 Rheumatoid factor positive by 3 months.
3 X-rays: erosions within 12 months.

Course and prognosis
The majority show protracted, active disease at 15 years review, with severe functional impairment in 30%.

Juvenile psoriatic arthritis

There is a family history in 40%.

Clinical features
1 M:F = 1:3; peak incidence of psoriasis at 10 years.
2 Joints: monoarticular 50%. Involvement of MCP, PIP and DIP in a single ray is common. The neck is affected in 10%.
3 Skin: psoriasis follows arthritis in 50%. It may start concurrently in 10% and nail pitting may be the sole manifestation.

Investigations
Sacroiliitis and spondylitis may occur late in the course in HLA B27 positive patients.

Course and prognosis
Prognosis is good for functional outcome, although disease may continue into adulthood.

Monarthritis

Aetiology
1 Trauma.
2 Mechanical derangement.
3 Infection.

5 Important rheumatological conditions

5.10 Paediatric rheumatology

4 Monoarticular presentation of polyarthritis.
5 blood dyscrasias.

Investigations
1 X-rays.
2 Synovial fluid microscopy and culture.
3 Synovial biopsy.
4 Arthroscopy (plant thorn synovitis).

5 Important rheumatological conditions

5.11 The vasculitides

- A heterogeneous group of disorders characterized by inflammatory changes occurring within the vessel wall causing vascular obliteration, infarction and haemorrhage.
- Clinical picture reflects site and size of vessel involvement.
- Underlying mechanisms are unknown and therefore the classification is unsatisfactory.
- Current grouping is according to clinicopathological criteria which has some bearing on prognosis.

Necrotizing vasculitis

A necrotizing vasculitis affecting small and medium sized arteries, which includes:
   polyarteritis nodosa (PAN);
   Kawasaki's disease;
   Churg–Strauss syndrome;
   Wegener's granulomatosis;
   vasculitis of connective tissue disease (e.g. RA, although there is much overlap).

Polyarteritis nodosa

This is typically restricted to small and medium sized arteries often with aneurysmal dilation. Infection with hepatitis B is an aetiological factor in some cases.

Clinical features
See Table 5.13.
1 Sex incidence equal; age of onset, middle-aged and elderly.
2 Initial manifestations non-specific reflecting systemic inflammation; later features depend on the distribution of affected arteries.
3 The occurrence of mononeuritis multiplex and fever is highly suggestive of PAN. Mononeuritis multiplex presents as simultaneous changes in several peripheral motor or sensory

5 Important rheumatological conditions

5.11 The vasculitides

Table 5.13. Clinical features of polyarteritis nodosa

> Fever 80%
> Disproportionate tachycardia 50%
> Weight loss
> Glomerulonephritis 70%
> Hypertension 70%
> Abdominal pain and diarrhoea
> Hepato 50%, splenomegaly 20%
> Testicular pain (20%)
> Mononeuritis multiplex 60%
> CNS involvement 40%
> Polyarthralgia 50%
> Rashes — livido reticularis
> Subcutaneous nodules along arteries (rare)

nerves, often as foot drop (popliteal nerve) with or without median/ulnar nerve involvement.

4 Predominantly cutaneous form in elderly.

Investigations
1 Urinalysis and microscopy of a fresh sample reveals microscopic haematuria and cellular casts.
2 ESR elevated with moderate normochromic normocytic anaemia and leucocytosis.
3 Abnormal LFTs 60%.
4 HBsAg 10% (USA 50%).
5 Immunological abnormalities unusual.
6 EMG and nerve conduction studies provide objective evidence of nerve and muscle involvement.
7 Biopsy of clinically involved tissue reveals muscle and sural nerve in mononeuritis multiplex and foot drop.
8 Renal, coeliac and mesenteric angiography: aneurysms occur at bifurcation of medium sized arteries. One or two small aneurysms are normal.

5 Important rheumatological conditions

5.11 The vasculitides

Differential diagnosis
A similar clinical picture is found in infective endocarditis and atrial myxoma.

Management
Specific diagnosis required as toxic, long-term therapy is required.
1 Symptomatic:
analgesics, NSAIDs;
treat hypertension;
splints for foot drop.
2 Specific — induction of remission. Owing to the difficulty in performing clinical trials in this rare condition various regimens are in use. One example is as follows: cyclophosphamide 2 mg/kg/ day and/or azathioprine 2.5 mg/kg/day with or without prednisolone EC 60–100 mg/day. Start to reduce steroids at 2 months if responding. Maintenance: oral prednisolone and low dose cyclophosphamide 100–150 mg/day.

Course and prognosis
This has improved: survival is 50% at 5 years and a cure has been reported. The main mortality is from renal, cardiac or CNS complications, although the cutaneous form in the elderly carries a good prognosis.

Kawasaki's disease (mucocutaneous lymph node syndrome)
This is a very rare childhood disorder, with most reported cases from Japan.

Clinical features
1 Predominantly males; children under 5 years.
2 Fever.
3 Hand oedema.
4 Skin: generalized macular erythematous rash, palms and soles with later desquamation of the finger tips. There are dry red lips

with a swollen strawberry tongue.
5 Conjunctivitis.
6 Lymphadenopathy.
7 Vasculitis affecting coronary arteries (95%), common iliacs (90%), superior mesenteric (85%), and abdominal aorta (80%).

Course and prognosis
Most patients recover although no specific treatment is available. There is 2% mortality due to vasculitis, myocarditis, ruptured aneurysms and conduction defects.

Churg–Strauss syndrome
The original cases were described by Churg and Strauss in 1951 and are now accepted as an entity separate from PAN. The histological appearance is of a necrotizing extravascular granulomatosis with vasculitis of small arteries and veins and an eosinophilic infiltrate.

Clinical features
1 Fever and weight loss.
2 Preceding atopic history (usually asthma) 100%; mean duration 8 years.
3 Rash 66%; tender subcutaneous nodules, palpable purpura.
4 Neurological involvement 60%; mononeuritis multiplex.
5 Abdominal pain 20%.
6 Polyarthralgia/arthritis 20%.
7 Renal disease 4%.

Investigations
1 Raised ESR with anaemia of chronic disease and eosinophilia.
2 Occasionally raised IgE.
3 CXR abnormal in 30% with transient patchy infiltrates, bilateral nodular infiltrates and diffuse interstitial disease.
4 Biopsy of muscle or involved tissue.

5 Important rheumatological conditions

5.11 The vasculitides

Management
Prednisolone EC 1 mg/kg/day, reduced according to clinical and laboratory findings.

Disease course and prognosis
There is a better prognosis than PAN, with 60% survival at 5 years.

Wegener's granulomatosis
This exhibits a dense mononuclear infiltrate with involvement of medium and small sized vessels. It is a triad of upper and lower respiratory tract disease with glomerulonephritis.

Clinical features
1. Respiratory system;
   pulmonary infiltrates 70%;
   cough;
   sinusitis;
   saddle nose deformity.
2. Arthralgia/arthritis 45%.
3. Glomerulonephritis 85%; 10% present in renal failure.
4. Serous otitis media 60%.
5. Eye involvement 60%; scleritis, proptosis.
6. Rash: papules, vesicles, purpura.
7. Neurological involvement 22%; cranial neuritis, mononeuritis multiplex.
8. Heart: pericarditis, coronary vasculitis.

Investigations
1. Urinalysis for haematuria and proteinuria with examination of fresh sediment for cellular casts.
2. Urea and electrolytes, creatinine clearance and protein excretion.
3. ESR raised with normochromic/normocytic anaemia and thrombocytosis in 20%.

4 Rheumatoid factor in 35%; ANF, HBsAg negative and antibodies to neutrophil alkaline phosphatase.
5 X-rays. Chest: multiple bilateral nodal infiltrates, some with cavitation; sinus: destructive changes.
6 Biopsy of lesion — nasopharynx, sinus, lung, kidney.

Management
Cyclophosphamide 2 mg/kg/day orally, prednisolone 1 mg/kg for 2–4 weeks then tailing. Maintain patient on cyclophosphamide at least 1 year following remission. Initial dose of cyclophosphamide may be doubled in life-threatening disease.

Disease course and prognosis
- Remission 90%.
- Relapses 25%.
- Eighty five per cent alive at 4 years.
- Deaths due to renal failure.

Vasculitis in connective tissue disease
Most commonly occurs in RA and SLE. In RA it is uncommon, but well recognized. All sizes of vessel may be involved.

The spectrum ranges from nailfold and digital vasculitis (relatively common: 14% M, 5% F), which is intermittent with no adverse prognostic implications, to PAN type, which is rare (<1%) and may be life-threatening and is a medical emergency.

Clinical features
1 Sex incidence equal: age of onset 60 years.
2 Usually long-standing; seropositive RA; synovitis often relatively inactive.
3 Peripheral sensory neuropathy 60%; mononeuritis multiplex 20% (poor prognosis).
4 Purpura 30%, punched out leg ulcers 30%, gangrene 15%.

5 Important rheumatological conditions

5.11 The vasculitides

Investigations
1 High ESR, anaemia.
2 High levels of rheumatoid factor with hypocomplementaemia.
3 Biopsy of muscle, sural nerve, skin and deep rectal mucosal (may be useful as a blind biopsy site).

Management
1 Digital and small vessel disease requires a second-line agent such as gold or penicillamine.
2 Severe vasculitis may only respond to a regime of pulsed intravenous cyclophosphamide and methyl prednisolone: day 1, cyclophosphamide 15 mg/kg i.v., methyl pred 1G i.v. (give over 30 min); day 8, repeat, according to response and FBC; at 2 weeks repeat, as above.

Note that there is no regime that has been adequately tested by appropriate randomized, double-blind trials. Hence all regimes are experimental. For further advice regarding these drugs see section 6.1.

Course and prognosis
Vasculitis is associated with an increased mortality in RA. Lone digital vasculitis has a good prognosis.

Small vessel vasculitis
This disease primarily involves the skin, with involvement of post capillary venules and capillaries with leucocytoclasis. It includes vasculitis following:
1 Infections:
   group A streptococci;
   Staphylococcus aureus;
   Neisseria gonorrhoea.
2 Drugs:
   sulphonamides;
   penicillin;
   thiazides;

5 Important rheumatological conditions

5.11 The vasculitides

allopurinol;
gold.
3 Malignancy:
carcinoma;
lymphoma.
4 Connective tissue diseases.
5 Henoch–Schönlein purpura.
6 Mixed essential cryoglobulinaemia.

Henoch–Schönlein purpura
This is sometimes caused by hypersensitivity or food allergy.

Clinical features
1 Age of onset 4–11, but can occur at any age.
2 Palpable purpura on lower extremities and buttocks.
3 Arthralgia/arthritis.
4 Glomerulonephritis.
5 Abdominal pain, occasionally intussusception.

Investigations
1 Throat swab to exclude streptococci.
2 Urinalysis and examination of urinary sediment.
3 Urine function tests.
4 Biopsy of skin, kidney; IgA deposition in skin and mesangium.

Management
There is no specific treatment. A prolonged follow-up is essential as hypertension or heavy proteinuria may develop years after original illness.

Disease course and prognosis
The prognosis is related to the presence of nephritis; 10% of these patients develop renal insufficiency.

5 Important rheumatological conditions

5.11 The vasculitides

Mixed essential cryoglobulinaemia

This condition is rare. The patient's serum contains a mixed IgG—IgM cryoglobulin complex with rheumatoid factor activity, which may be associated with HBsAg in 66%.

Clinical features
1 Females predominant (2:1); age of onset > 50 years.
2 Purpura 85%, especially over lower extremities.
3 Arthralgias 50%.
4 Renal involvement: proteinuria 50%, renal failure 45%, hypertension 40%.
5 Splenomegaly 45%
6 Raynaud's 30%.
7 Neurological involvement; parasthaesiae 12.5%, foot drop 7.5%.

Investigations
1 Urinalysis and examination of fresh urinary sediment for cellular casts.
2 Renal function tests.
3 FBC: anaemia common.
4 Liver function tests.
5 HBsAg.
6 Cryoglobulins (cold precipitating immunoglobulins). These are detected by allowing the blood to clot at 37°C. The warm serum is removed and stored at 4°C for 72 h.
7 Rheumatoid factor usually elevated with hypocomplementaemia.
8 Biopsy of skin and kidney.

Management
1 Prednisolone EC 1 mg/kg/day.
2 Cyclophosphamide 2 mg/kg/day.
3 Plasmapheresis.

5 Important rheumatological conditions

5.11 The vasculitides

Course and prognosis
This is mainly determined by the presence of renal disease. It is fatal in 70% with renal disease, 30% without.

Giant cell vasculitis

In this condition the large arteries are involved. It is a panarteritis with mononuclear infiltrate and disruption of the internal elastic lamina and giant cells. It includes: giant cell arteritis and Takayasu's arteritis.

Giant cell arteritis
See section 7.6.

Takayasu's arteritis
This condition is rare. It has a worldwide distribution, but is more common in the Orient.

Clinical features
1 Predominantly females; 20−50 years.
2 Pre-pulseless symptoms precede pulse deficits by months:
   fatigue 70%;
   exertional dyspnoea 45%;
   headaches 50%;
   arthralgias 50%;
   myalgia 40%;
   weight loss 20%;
   fever 15%;
   transient rashes 15%.
3 Late pulseless symptoms reflect site of arterial involvement:
   arterial bruits 80%;
   hypertension 60%;
   claudication 45%;
   congestive cardiac failure 35%;
   visual disturbances 15%;
   syncope 10%;

Raynaud's 9%;
abdominal pain 9%.

Investigations
1 ESR, CRP markedly raised with hypochromic, normocytic anaemia.
2 X-rays: AXR shows post-stenotic dilation of the aorta. Arteriography is diagnostic.

Management
1 Prednisolone EC 30 mg/day for 9 weeks; maintenance dose 5–10 mg for 6 months.
2 ESR is the best monitor of disease activity.
3 Treat hypertension and heart failure as necessary.
4 Consider vascular surgery in the symptomatic, chronic stage.

Disease course and prognosis
There is an indolent disease course with a 5-year survival of 85%.

5 Important rheumatological conditions

5.12 Rarer rheumatic syndromes

5.12 Rarer rheumatic syndromes

Adult Still's disease
This disease occurs between 20 and 35 years.

Symptoms
- High fever.
- Sore throat.
- Pain in wrists, knees and fingers.
- Rash.
- Chest pain, abdominal pain.

Signs
- Quotidian fever.
- Polyarthritis of above joints.
- Evanescent rash, most apparent when patients are febrile; salmon pink, macular rash with the trunk predominantly involved but also arms and legs including palms and soles.
- Serositis; pericarditis 20%, pleural effusions.
- Lymphadenopathy, mesenteric adenitis.
- Hepatomegaly, splenomegaly 33%.

Investigations
- X-ray: erosive ankylosis of PIP and DIP joints, sparing of MCP joints with carpal and cervical spine ankylosis.
- Blood: raised ESR, CRP, leucocytosis 97%, anaemia 88%, abnormal liver function tests 80%, latex, ANF negative, ASO titre normal.

Treatment and prognosis
NSAIDs and steroids for systemic disease. It is a self-limiting disorder in 40%, with 60% of patients showing persistent disease activity. Amyloidosis may occur in a few.

5 Important rheumatological conditions

5.12 Rarer rheumatic syndromes

Amyloidosis
1 Primary and myeloma-associated — AL amyloid.
2 Secondary to chronic disease — AA amyloid, e.g. rheumatoid arthritis, juvenile chronic arthritis, TB, leprosy, bronchiectasis, hypernephroma, Hodgkin's disease.
3 Heredofamilial amyloidoses.

Symptoms (primary amyloid)
- Malaise, early morning stiffness.
- Pains in shoulders, wrists, knees and fingers.
- Enlargement of the tongue.
- Paraesthesiae of the extremities.
- Shortness of breath.

Signs
- Synovitis affecting large and small joints.
- 'Shoulder-pad' sign: glenohumeral joint involvement with amyloid.
- Subcutaneous nodules 50%.
- Waxy plaques around the axilla, anal, inguinal regions.
- Malaena from haemorrhagic diathesis.
- Macroglossia, hepatospenomegaly.
- Peripheral and autonomic neuropathy.
- Carpal tunnel syndrome.
- Congestive cardiac failure.
- Non-thrombocytopenic purpura.

Investigations
X-rays show soft tissue swelling; erosions are uncommon. The echocardiogram indicates restrictive cardiomyopathy. Laboratory findings show latex occasionally positive and there may be evidence of nephrotic syndrome. Tissue biopsy from rectum, skin, gingiva and subcutaneous abdominal fat, on Congo Red staining, shows apple green birefringence.

5 Important rheumatological conditions

5.12 Rarer rheumatic syndromes

Treatment and prognosis
Chemotherapy is needed if there is associated myeloma. No specific treatment is available for amyloid deposits and prognosis is generally poor (renal failure, cardiac arrythmias). Dental extraction is necessary if tongue ulceration threatens.

Behçet's syndrome
This is a rare condition in Europe, being more common in Eastern Mediterranean countries and Japan. There is a male predominance (2:1), age 18–40 years.

Symptoms
- Mouth ulcers 98% — recurrent, very painful.
- Genital ulcers 80%.
- Abdominal pain.
- Eye problems.
- Joint pain 30–60%.
- Neurological symptoms (most common in Japan).
- Tender skin nodules.

Signs
- Oral ulcers involve lips, gums, palate, posterior pharynx with punched out or with central grey membrane.
- Genital ulcers may affect scrotum, glans penis, vulva, vagina and cervix.
- Tender abdomen, intestinal perforation, intestinal ulcers may simulate Crohn's disease.
- Uveitis 80%: anterior and more commonly posterior with conjunctivitis, scleritis, retinal vasculitis and optic neuritis also seen.
- Polyarthritis: knees, ankles, less often wrists affected; chronic, non-migratory, non-destructive; sacroiliitis and spondylitis may occur.
- Transient episodes of brain stem dysfunction, also meningoencephalitis, pseudotumour cerebri, cranial nerve

5 Important rheumatological conditions

5.12 Rarer rheumatic syndromes

palsies, confusional states progressing to dementia.
- Thrombophlebitis 30%
- Skin hypersensitivity — aseptic pustule develops at site of venepuncture after 24−48 h.

Investigations
No characteristic laboratory findings.

Management
1 NSAIDs for arthritis.
2 Colchicine may reduce the frequency of ulcerative lesions.
3 Lignocaine gel may help oral ulcers.
4 Ocular lesions respond best to cyclophosphamide or chlorambucil.
5 Steroids may worsen prognosis in ocular or CNS disease.

Familial Mediterranean fever
This condition affects Mediteranean peoples, especially Sephardic and Iraqi Jews. It is an autosomal recessive inheritance, with a sex incidence $M:F = 3:2$. Onset occurs in childhood and adolescence.

Symptoms
There are recurrent attacks of fever and joint pains, especially knees, also ankles, hips and shoulders with sometimes abdominal or chest pain.

Signs
- Fever.
- Pain and disability disproportionate to joint signs.
- Asymmetrical oligoarthritis.
- Splenomegaly.
- Abdominal crises may simulate peritonitis.

5 Important rheumatological conditions

5.12 Rarer rheumatic syndromes

Investigations
X-rays are usually normal but osteoporosis and pseudocysts are reported with prolonged attacks. There is widening or sclerosis of SI joints reported.
 Blood: ESR normal or raised. Leucocytosis common.

Treatment and prognosis
Analgesics and NSAIDs are indicated. Colchicine (0.5 mg b.d.) prevents attacks. Prognosis is good, but AA amyloidosis may develop in 30%.

Hyperlipoproteinaemia
This occurs with hyperbetalipoproteinaemia (Friedrickson's Type II) and hypertriglyceridaemia (Friedrickson's Type IV).
1 Hyperbetalipoproteinaemia is an autosomal dominant inherited disorder of cholesterol metabolism; 18% have arthritis on presentation, 50% after 4 years. M=F, often presents in childhood.
2 Hypertriglyceridaemia may be inherited (autosomal dominant) and may be secondary to hypothyroidism, nephrotic syndrome. It is exacerbated by obesity and alcohol. M=F, onset 40–60 years.

Symptoms
There is early morning stiffness and episodic polyarthralgias.

Signs
Joint swelling, erythema with loss of function and Achilles tendinitis may occur, as well as xanthomata.

Investigations
X-ray is usually normal, although erosion of phalanges may occur. Para-articular bone cysts occur with hypertriglyceridaemia.
 Blood: raised serum cholesterol (hyperbetalipoproteinaemia), elevated triglycerides, cholesterol normal or slightly raised (hypertriglyceridaemia).

5 Important rheumatological conditions

5.12 Rarer rheumatic syndromes

Treatment and prognosis
This is dependent on diet and NSAIDs.

In hyperbetalipoproteinaemia, use cholesterol lowering agents, e.g. cholestyramine 8 g b.d., 1, colestipol 10 mg b.d., and probucol 500 mg b.d. There should be screening of other family members. Prognosis is related to the high incidence of premature ischaemic heart disease.

In hypertriglyceridaemia, increase proportion of polyunsaturated fatty acids in diet, instigate weight reduction and reduce alcohol intake. Administer nicotinic acid.

Hypermobility

This condition may be idiopathic or secondary to various inheritable diseases:
  Marfan's syndrome;
  Ehlers–Danlos;
  osteogenesis imperfecta (mild forms);
  homocystinuria.

Onset in childhood occurs as an effusion or in adults as premature OA (30–40 years). M=F.

Symptoms
Knee pain is commonest (20%), but also small joints of hands and wrists. There is a history of being 'double-jointed'.

Signs
- Hypermobility (see section 1.2 for Beighton scoring system).
- Joint effusions.
- Bony swelling and crepitus.

Investigations
X-rays are normal early on, but features of OA develop later. Blood is normal.

5 Important rheumatological conditions

5.12 Rarer rheumatic syndromes

Treatment and prognosis
Treatment is symptomatic and prognosis is good.

Hypertrophic pulmonary osteoarthropathy
This is defined as:
proliferative periostitis of long bones;
clubbing;
synovitis.

It may be primary and is usually inherited, e.g. pachydermoperiostosis (autosomal dominant inheritance, leonine facies, greasy skin, clubbing, recurrent joint effusions, mild joint pain)

If it is secondary, features include:
chronic suppurative pulmonary disease;
bronchogenic carcinoma;
congenital cyanotic heart disease;
bacterial endocarditis;
cirrhosis;
inflammatory bowel disease;
thyroid acropachy.

The clinical features of the secondary form may precede features of underlying disease by up to 18 months.

Symptoms
- Insidious onset.
- Severe pain of distal limbs.
- Exacerbated by dependency, relieved by elevation of limb.
- Symmetrical pains of many joints: MCPJs, wrists, elbows, knees, ankles.

Signs
There is clubbing, warm, tender joints with effusions and warm distal extremities.

5 Important rheumatological conditions

5.12 Rarer rheumatic syndromes

Investigations
X-ray shows periosteal elevation along shaft of long bones (Fig. 5.24). Bone scanning indicates increased uptake along long bone shafts, phalanges ('string of lights' appearance). CXR may reveal evidence of lung malignancy.

Treatment and prognosis
- NSAIDs are indicated.
- Vagotomy, tumour resection.
- Prognosis is of underlying condition.

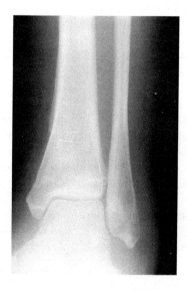

Fig. 5.24 Hypertrophic pulmonary osteoarthrophathy showing diaphyseal periostial reaction. Note lack of involvement of metaphysis and former epiphysis.

Intermittent hydrarthrosis
An idiopathic, cyclic recurrence of joint effusions with complete

5 Important rheumatological conditions

5.12 Rarer rheumatic syndromes

freedom from signs and symptoms between attacks. F:M = 3:1 with peak age of onset 20–30 years.

Symptoms
There is pain, stiffness and swelling of one or two joints. The knee is the most commonly affected; the only joint involved in 60%. Others include elbow, hip, shoulder, ankle and tempero-mandibular joint. Swelling occurs regularly — usually every 1–2 weeks.

Signs
Large cool effusions, occasionally fever.

Investigations
X-rays: soft tissue swelling only. Blood: normal tests. Synovial fluid is non-inflammatory.

Treatment and prognosis
Conservative management only. Aspiration and steroid injections are of short-term benefit only. Synovectomy may be considered if severe, although there is recurrence in 50%. In the long term 54% resolve, 32% continue, 14% milder, less frequent attacks. There is no joint damage.

Multicentric reticulohistiocytosis
This is an erosive nodular arthritis often resembling rheumatoid arthritis, with mean age 43 (11–71), M:F=3:1.

Symptoms
There is pain and swelling of large and small joints, occasionally fever and weight loss and tiny skin nodules appear later.

Signs
- Symmetrical polyarthritis in distribution similar to RA, except DIP involvement more common.

5   Important rheumatological conditions

5.12   Rarer rheumatic syndromes

- Arthritis mutilans 40–50%.
- Nodules around ears, nose, neck, nailfolds and mucosal membranes.
- Xanthelasma 30%.
- Malignancy 20–30%.

Investigations
X-ray shows surface and cystic erosions around joints, including the DIP joints. Blood: ESR elevated, latex negative. Biopsy of nodule shows foamy, multinucleate giant cells filled with PAS positive material.

Treatment and prognosis
Use NSAIDs; if severe, consider immunosuppressive agents. Disease course may be progressive and destructive.

Pigmented villonodular synovitis
A benign synovial proliferation causing grape-like villi. Onset in the third decade, M=F.

Symptoms
There is insidious onset of pain and swelling in one, sometimes two, joints, usually the knee, 80%; others include hip, foot, ankles, finger tendon sheaths, elbows and rarely wrist or shoulders.

Signs
There is synovial thickening; joint may be warm with blood-stained effusion.

Investigations
X-ray: soft tissue opacity. There may be juxta-articular osteoporosis and cystic erosions. Arthroscopy and synovial biopsy are diagnostic.

5 Important rheumatological conditions

5.12 Rarer rheumatic syndromes

Treatment and prognosis
There is a chronic course with acute episodes and synovectomy recurs in 30%.

Plant thorn synovitis
A synovitis caused by unnoticed penetration of the joint by plant thorn (UK), or cactus spine (USA).

Symptoms
There is an initial episode of pain and swelling of the knee (children) or finger (gardeners) which resolves, with recurrent intermittent joint swelling thereafter.

Signs
A monoarthritis with effusion and synovial thickening. There may be flexion contracture and occasionally fever.

Investigations
X-ray is normal or shows small bony erosions. Blood: raised ESR. Synovial fluid is inflammatory and on synovial biopsy thorn fragments are visible especially on polarized light microscopy with chronic granulomatous reaction around thorn.

Treatment and prognosis
Synovectomy is curative; otherwise chronic intermittent arthritis if undiagnosed.

Rheumatic fever
This is a condition of carditis, arthritis, chorea and erythema marginatum with evidence of preceding Group A β-haemolytic streptococcal infection. M=F, onset 5–15 years. 80% have arthritis.

Symptoms
There is preceding sore throat 2–3 weeks earlier, then an acute

onset with flitting migratory joint pains, usually starting in the lower limbs proceeding to the arms. Course is altered by antibiotics; may stay in one or two joints.

Signs
Joints are tender and swollen; often pain is more prominent than objective signs would suggest. There are firm, non-tender, subcutaneous nodules (10%). Chorea (10%) disappears on sleep, may occur at rest. Carditis in 10% (pericarditis 5–10%, conduction changes) and valve lesions especially mitral with mid-diastolic (Carey Coombs) murmur. Erythema marginatum in 20%.

Investigations
- X-ray shows joints normal and CXR exhibits cardiomegaly in 20%.
- Blood: ESR elevated. ASO titre raised in 80% (peaks 4–5 weeks following sore throat). The rest have elevation of one or more other antibodies including anti-DNAase and antihyaluronidase.
- Throat swab shows β-haemolytic streptococcus, Lancefield Group A.
- ECG: prolonged PR interval.

Treatment and prognosis
- Bed rest, NSAIDs, penicillin plus the treatment of complications. Regular chemoprophylaxis is not required, but intercurrent throat infections should be treated promptly with penicillin.
- Average duration of the rheumatic attack is 3 weeks, <5% persist more than 6 months.
- Prognosis is worse if there is carditis in the initial attack. Jaccoud's arthropathy may develop in a few (ulnar deviation, flexion of MCP joints, hyperextension of PIPJs, hook-like erosions on hand X-ray).

5 Important rheumatological conditions

5.12 Rarer rheumatic syndromes

Neuropathic joint disease (Charcot's joints)
This condition exhibits joint failure secondary to neuropathy. Causes and main joints affected include:
  diabetes—tarsal and tarso-metatarsals;
  syringomyelia—shoulders;
  tabes dorsalis—knee, ankles, hip, spine;
  Riley—Day syndrome;
  congenital indifference to pain—all joints in young people;
  leprosy—small joints of hands and feet;
  yaws—as in tabes;
  Charcot—Marie—Tooth syndrome—ankle subtaloids;
  spinal cord and peripheral nerve lesions—corresponds to nerves damaged;
  familial sensory neuropathy—joints of feet.

Symptoms
Pain is seldom completely absent, since skin and neighbouring nerve territories may remain pain sensitive. Foot deformities cause painful shoe pressures. Acute swelling or inflammation may distend skin. Clinically, the joint damage is out of proportion to the pain and loss of function. 'Lightning' pain occurs in tabes.

Signs
An acute onset presents with warm, swollen joints; in chronic disease large effusions are common. There is joint instability, crepitus and an insensitive joint capsule on joint aspiration.

Investigations
- X-ray shows:
  soft tissue swelling;
  multiple loose bodies—fragments of bone and calcified cartilage;
  disorganized joint;
  marked osteophytosis;
  juxta-articular sclerosis;
  joint fractures and deformity.

5 Important rheumatological conditions

5.12 Rarer rheumatic syndromes

- Blood shows:
  ESR normal;
  VDRL and TPI tests for syphilis.
- Synovial fluid is non-inflammatory and often blood-stained.

Treatment and prognosis
Bed rest for acute arthritis, joint splinting and surgery for severe instability. The prognosis is generally a gradual progression.

Relapsing polychondritis
An episodic inflammatory disorder of cartilage which affects:
  external ears;
  nose;
  respiratory tract;
  joints;
  heart valves;
  eyes.
M=F, onset 40–60 years.

Symptoms
- Pain and stiffness of large and small joints (80%).
- Parasternal articulations may also be involved.
- Abrupt onset of pain in the nose or external ear.
- Vertigo or hearing difficulty.
- Acutely painful eye.
- Breathing difficulty.

Signs
- Asymmetrical joint swelling occurs with limitation of movement.
- Inflamed tender nose leading to saddle nose deformity.
- Swollen inflamed pinnae.
- Cochlear and vestibular dysfunction.

5 Important rheumatological conditions

5.12 Rarer rheumatic syndromes

- Iritis, scleritis.
- Hoarseness, stridor.
- Incompetence of heart valves; aortic > mitral, tricuspid.

Investigations
X-ray shows normal joints, or juxta-articular osteoporosis, whilst CXR or CT scan exhibits tracheal stenosis.
  Blood: raised ESR with anaemia and leucocytosis.
  Cartilage biopsy is diagnostic.

Treatment and prognosis
- NSAIDs.
- Corticosteroids 30–60 mg/day; dapsone 50–200 mg/day has been used.
- Cytotoxic agents and corticosteroids with tracheal involvement.
- Variable clinical course: usually episodic flares, may be fulminant.
- Tracheal and cardiovascular involvement indicate poor prognosis.

Sarcoid arthropathy
Two forms of arthropathy occur with sarcoidosis: an acute variety associated with erythema nodosum and bilateral hilar adenopathy (Löfgren's syndrome); and a more chronic form associated with multi-organ sarcoidosis.
  Sarcoidosis may also produce bony lesions (osseous sarcoid).

Löfgren's syndrome — symptoms
- F:M = 3:1.
- Abrupt onset of migratory joint pain (75%) affecting ankles, knees, wrists, PIP joints, elbows.
- Painful raised lumps over limbs (lower > upper).
- Malaise, fever.

5 Important rheumatological conditions

5.12 Rarer rheumatic syndromes

Signs
- Symmetrical polyarthritis, tenosynovitis and periarthritis.
- Erythema nodosum.
- Fever in 37%.

Investigations
- X-ray shows soft tissue swelling, whilst CXR exhibits bihilar adenopathy.
- Blood: raised ESR, latex test is positive in 15–40% with hyperuricaemia in 25%.

Treatment and prognosis
NSAIDs, prednisolone. Colchicine may shorten acute attacks. The majority have a single attack lasting 2–4 weeks and there is an excellent prognosis.

Chronic and osseous form

Clinical features
- Usually recurrent episodes of oligo/monoarthritis, which occasionally affects multiple joints and is destructive.
- Active systemic sarcoidosis.
- Skin lesions are common with bone involvement, e.g. lupus pernio.
- Swollen fingers (dactylitis).

Investigations
- X-rays: bone lesions show osteolytic lesions and a lacey trabecular pattern (Fig. 5.25).
- Blood: urinary and serum calcium, hypercalcuria early sign.
- Biopsy of skin lesion.
- Kveim test: 0.2 ml of 10% saline suspension of sarcoid tissue given intradermally. Mark injection site and take skin biopsy 6 weeks later.
- Gallium scanning.

5 Important rheumatological conditions

5.12 Rarer rheumatic syndromes

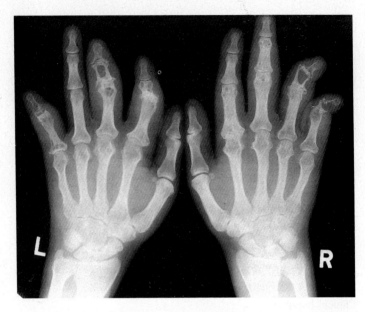

Fig. 5.25 Sarcoid dactylitis showing soft tissue swelling, multiple central lytic lesions with bone destruction and lacey trabeculation in undestroyed bone (L proximal phalanx).

Treatment
Lessions may resolve with corticosteroids and some success has been reported with use of methotrexate and azathioprine.

Sweet's syndrome
A febrile illness associated with skin nodules, arthritis and leucocytosis with an histological appearance of dense neutrophil dermal infiltrate which is characteristic. F=M, onset 35–50 years.

Symptoms
Twenty-five per cent have joint symptoms, commonly affecting

5 Important rheumatological conditions

5.12 Rarer rheumatic syndromes

hands, wrists, ankles and knees. There are painful skin nodules with low grade fever, fatigue and malaise.

Signs
Symmetrical polyarthritis. Raised, tender purple plaques on face, neck and limbs which resolve without scarring in 2−3 months.

Investigations
- X-ray is normal. Blood shows raised ESR, CRP with leucocytosis.
- Skin biopsy shows dense dermal infiltration with mature polymorphonucleocytes.

6 Therapy

6.1 Drug therapy, 239

6.2 Rehabilitation, 256

6.3 Surgery, 262

6.4 Chiropody and shoe prescription, 268

6.5 Diet in arthritis, 272

6 Therapy

6.1 Drug therapy

6.1 Drug therapy

Non-steroidal anti-inflammatory drugs (NSAIDs)
There are 22 preparations of NSAIDs listed in the current British National Formulary (Table 6.1). They owe their anti-inflammatory properties to their ability to inhibit the enzyme cyclo-oxygenase, which takes part in the conversion of arachidonic acid to prostaglandins, which are essential mediators of inflammation.

Pharmacology
NSAIDs are absorbed rapidly from the gastro-intestinal tract and mainly metabolized in the liver. In body fluids they are extensively, though reversibly, protein bound. As a group, they are acidic and lipid soluble, so that the rate of renal elimination is increased in an alkaline urine. Sulindac and fenbufen are 'pro-drugs', inactive as swallowed, but converted to an active form in the liver. Controlled clinical trials seldom distinguish the available preparations in efficacy.

Toxicity (Table 6.2)

Upper gastrointestinal tract. Local irritation: NSAIDs may irritate the gastric lining by direct contact.

Systemic effects: the mucous membrane of the stomach is protected against digestive acids and enzymes by secretion of bicarbonate into the mucus barrier and by the regulation of local blood flow. These protective mechanisms are mediated by prostaglandin E_2 and hence reduced by the cyclo-oxygenase inhibiting effects of NSAIDs.

Adverse effects include: mild heartburn, anaemia from gastrointestinal erosion (micro-bleeding), acute gastrointestinal ulceration and perforation.

Colon. The fenamates tend to cause diarrhoea. All NSAIDs should be prescribed with caution in patients with chronic inflammatory bowel disease.

Table 6.1. NSAIDs – dosage and adverse effects (modified from Dieppe et al. 1985).

Drug	Dose	Common	Less common	Comments
Diclofenac	50 mg t.d.s. or 100 mg nocte (supp) 100 mg SR o.d.	GID, headache, dizziness	Rash, oedema	Safe with AC Not detectable in breast milk
Indomethacin	25 mg t.d.s. 75 mg (SR) nocte/b.d. 100 mg nocte (supp)	GID, headache, confusion	Oedema, peripheral neuropathy	Avoid in elderly due to oedema CNS effect
Sulindac	200 mg b.d.	GID	Rash, CNS disturbance, raised LFT's	A prodrug Safe with AC
Tolmetin	400 mg t.d.s./q.d.s.	GID, CNS	Rash, oedema	Safe with AC
Aspirin	600–900 mg 6/day	GID, hearing		Toxicity is frequent
Aloxiprin	1200 mg q.d.s.	Drug displacement and interaction		
Benorylate	Tabs 1.5 g t.d.s.	Hypersensitivity tinnitus and renal effects		EC preparation better tolerated. NB Benorylate contains aspirin and paracetamol
Salsalate	500 mg–1 g b.d.	Hepatitis		
Diflunisal	250–500 mg b.d.			
Fenbufen	600 mg nocte ± 300 mg o.d.	GID, rash		A prodrug Aspirin reduces drug levels by

Drug	Dose	Side effects		Notes
Fenoprofen	500–600 mg q.d.s.	GID	Rash	
Flurbiprofen	50–100 mg t.d.s.	GID	Rash	
Ibuprofen	300–600 mg q.d.s.	GID	Rash	
Ketoprofen	50–100 mg b.d. 100–200 mg o.d. (SR) 100 mg o.d. (supp)	GID	Rash	
Naproxen	250–500 mg b.d.	GID	Rash	
Mefanamic acid	500 mg t.d.s.	Diarrhoea, rash	Haemolysis	
Azapropazone	600 mg b.d.	GID Uricosuric. Induces microsomal enzymes	Rash, oedema Occ haemolysis	Requires adequate fluid intake
Phenylbutazone	100 mg q.d.s.	GID, rash, oedema	Hepatitis, goitre	Only for ankylosing spondylitis; restricted to prescription by hospital consultant
Piroxicam	20 mg o.d.	GID	Oedema, rash	

GID = gastrointestinal disease, AC = anticoagulants, supp = suppositories, SR = slow release preparation.

6 Therapy

6.1 Drug therapy

Table 6.2. Non-steroidal anti-inflammatory drugs — generic (bold type) and proprietary names

Substituted carboxylic acids

Salicylic acids
- **Aspirin**
  - Solprin
  - Paynocil
  - Nu-seals
  - Onadox
  - Levius
  - Laboprin
  - Hypon
  - Codis
  - Antoin
  - Breoprin
  - Caprin
  - Claradin
- **Aloxiprin**
  - Palaprin
- **Benorylate**
  - Benoral
- **Diflunisal**
  - Dolobid
- **Salsalate**
  - Disalcid
- **Choline Magnesium Trisalicylate**
  - Trilisate

Propionic acids
- **Fenbufen**
  - Lederfen
- **Fenoprofen**
  - Progesic
  - Fenopron
- **Flurbiprofen**
  - Froben

Propionic acids (cont.)
- **Ibuprofen**
  - Brufen
  - Ebufac
  - Ibu-slo
  - Apsifen
  - Fenbid
  - Lidifen
  - Motrin
  - Paxofen
- **Ketoprofen**
  - Orudis
  - Alrheumat
- **Naproxen**
  - Naprosyn
  - Napsalgesic
  - Synflex
  - Laraflex
- **Tiaproaenic acid**
  - Surgam
- **Suprofen**
  - Suprol

Fenamic acids
- **Mefenamic acid**
  - Ponstan

6 Therapy

6.1 Drug therapy

Table 6.2. (cont)

Benzotriazene
Azapropazone
Rheumox

Enolic acids
Pyrazolones
Feprazone
Methrazone

Phenylbutazone
Butazolidin
Parazoliadin
Butacote

Oxicams
Piroxicam
Feldene
Larapam

Tenoxicam
Imadyl

Phenylacetic acids
Diclofenac
Voltarol
Rhumalgen

Carbo and heterocyclic acetic acids
Indomethacin
Imbrilon
Indocid
Mobilan
Artracin
Indolar
Nadoflex
Indoflex
Rheumacin
Flexin Continus
Sulindac

Alkamone
Nabumetone
Relifex

Pyranocarboxylic acids
Etodolac
Lodine
Ramodar

Renal. NSAIDs should be used with caution in those with impaired renal function, congestive cardiac failure, hepatic failure with ascites and in the elderly. Combinations with angiotensin convertase inhibitors may cause a sharp deterioration in renal function. Other reported toxicity includes acute interstitial nephritis, reversible on stopping the drug, renal papillary necrosis, nephrotic syndrome and hyperkalaemia.

6 Therapy

6.1 Drug therapy

Skin. Macular or confluent erythemata. The Stevens–Johnson syndrome has been described with sulindac and diclofenac.

Central nervous system. Indomethacin in sufficient dosage causes 'muzziness', headache, confusion and occasionally hallucinations. The elderly are at special risk.

Cardiovascular. NSAIDs have weak fluid retaining activity. They may exacerbate heart failure and antagonize the effect of diuretics and anti-hypertensive therapy.

Respiratory. Caution is needed with patients with known aspirin-induced asthma or urticaria.

Indications
NSAIDs are widely prescribed and now available in over-the-counter preparations. However, serious toxicity may occur in patients on the drug for doubtful indications.
  Positive indications are: inflammatory arthropathies such as rheumatoid arthritis, ankylosing spondilitis and Reiter's syndrome.
  Relative indications are: osteoarthritis (restrict to inflammatory exacerbations) and soft tissue rheumatism (short periods only).

What to do in special circumstances

Minor gastrointestinal bleeding. Endoscopy is mandatory and the offending drug should be withdrawn.
  If NSAID is necessary (patient with active rheumatoid arthritis) change to a prodrug or another class of drug.
  Give ulcer healing advice (stop smoking) and give gastro-protective drugs such as tripotassium dicitro bismuthate or sucralfate or histamine II receptor antagonists (especially with duodenal ulcerations or misoprostol).
  Repeat endoscopy in 2 months. A number of studies have

shown that continuing NSAID therapy does not retard ulcer healing.

The presence or absence of indigestion is no safeguard as to whether gastrointestinal ulceration is till present or has healed.

Concurrent anticoagulant therapy. Competition for protein-binding may displace anticoagulants and increase their action. This can be compensated for by adjusting the dose of anticoagulant according to the prothrombin time.

Long-acting disease modifying agents
These have been shown in clinical trials to induce remissions in many patients with rheumatoid arthritis. There is a delay of 6 weeks or more between starting treatment and improvement or between stopping treatment and relapse. The indications for their prescription in rheumatoid arthritis have been set out previously (section 5.1).

Antimalarials
Hydroxychloroquine is the main drug of this class.

Indications
Rheumatoid arthritis, systemic lupus erythematosus.

Dose
200 mg twice a day for 1 year, after which the dose may be halved. Disease remission may be delayed for up to 3 months, but relapses on withdrawal or premature reduction of dose are common.

Monitoring
Ophthalmological referral on commencement of drug and then yearly or according to ophthalmologist.

6 Therapy

6.1 Drug therapy

Adverse effects
Hydroxychloroquine has low toxicity. Major concern is maculopathy which is very rare, but requires monitoring by ophthalmologist. Other toxicity includes diarrhoea, rashes which can be photosensitive, headaches, giddiness and myopathy.

Cautions
Should not be used in patients with psoriasis as it may exacerbate the rash.

Gold

Parenteral
Sodium aurothiomalate is given as an intramuscular injection.

Indications
Rheumatoid arthritis — experience suggests that this can be an effective agent in those patients who tolerate it. Adverse reactions occur in 30% and together with lack of response and non-compliance, not more than 50% of patients started on gold are still taking it at the end of 1 year.

Dose
Test doses of 5 mg, 20 mg are given with at least 2-day spacing. If no sensitivity reactions occur, the full dose of 50 mg per week for 12 weeks is prescribed, followed by 50 mg monthly for at least a year.

Thereafter, patients who respond to and tolerate gold injections should continue indefinitely perhaps on 'trickle' dosage of 20 mg monthly or 50 mg 2-monthly. The dosage may be increased up to 50 mg monthly during disease and then reduced as a response is obtained.

Stopping gold on improvement is followed by relapse and second courses are not as effective.

6 Therapy

6.1 Drug therapy

Monitoring
2-weekly full blood count and urinalysis for the first month, then monthly. The patient is told to report any rash.

Adverse effects
1 Rash — occasionally progresses to an exfoliative dermatitis and stomatitis. Since mild, non-specific rashes, unrelated to gold are common, it is important to see the rash since if unrelated, it may not entail stopping the treatment.
2 Proteinuria — may progress to nephrotic syndrome as a result of membranous glomerulonephritis. It usually recovers after 12–18 months. More than 1 g per 24 h should suggest drug withdrawal. Simple proteinuria is compatible with complete recovery of renal function.
3 Bone marrow toxicity — thrombocytopenia and pancytopenia rarely occurs early in treatment. Thrombocytopenia is preceded by a gradual reduction of the count over several months before serious depletion occurs. Bone marrow aspiration is needed to confirm the diagnosis. Penicillamine by mouth and dimercaprol (BAL) by injection will increase the removal of gold.
4 Others — common are vasomotor symptoms at time of injection, such as weakness, giddiness and sweating. In up to 15% transient stiffness, myalgias, may occur related to the injection. Acute hepatitis, patchy pulmonary consolidation, enterocolitis are rare.

Oral
Auranofin is better tolerated than parenteral gold and is four times less likely to be withdrawn. However, it may be less efficacious.

Dose
3 mg b.d.

Monitoring
As with parental gold.

6 Therapy

6.1 Drug therapy

Adverse effects
Rash and thrombocytopenia occur half as often as with parenteral gold, but dermatitis and albuminuria occur as often. Diarrhoea is often dose-related and responds to dose reduction.

Penicillamine

Indications
Rheumatoid arthritis — penicillamine has become one of the most important second-line drugs.

Dose
125 mg daily, increasing every 6 weeks to 375 mg or until an effect is obtained. The dose may be increased to 750 mg and even to 1 g in individual patients, although toxic effects are more common with the higher dosages. Up to 3 months treatment may be required before benefit is shown.

Penicillamine should be taken first thing in the morning at least 1 hour before breakfast and 4 hours away from any iron-containing preparations that reduce absorption of penicillamine.

Monitoring
2-weekly full blood count and urinalysis for first month, then monthly.

Adverse effects
1 Thrombocytopenia and, less commonly, neutropenia. Withdraw drug if white cell count falls below 3×10^9/l or platelet count less than 100×10^9/l. A downward trend within the normal range should be watched with caution. Once the blood count has returned to normal it may be possible to reintroduce the drug at a lower dose. However, if further evidence of marrow suppression occurs then the drug should be withdrawn permanently. Deaths from aplastic anaemia have been reported.
2 Proteinuria is relatively common, occurring in up to 30%.

6 Therapy

6.1 Drug therapy

Proteinuria greater than 2 g per 24 h should lead to drug withdrawal or dosage reduction. Biopsies show a membranous glomerulonephritis (reversible).

3 Rashes are often transient and respond to dosage reduction. Pemphigus has been described. Mouth ulcers are fairly common and may be severe. It is important to check the blood count in patients on penicillamine with mouth ulcers to exclude an underlying neutropenia.

4 Others: taste disturbance is common within the first 3 months and usually resolves spontaneously without changing the dose of drug. Autoimmune diseases such as Goodpasture's syndrome, polymyositis, myasthenia gravis, systemic lupus erythematosus and Sjögren's syndrome occur rarely.

Sulphasalazine

Sulphasalazine is a compound of sulphapyridine and para-amino salicylic acid. The drug is probably less toxic but also less effective than gold and penicillamine.

Indications
Rheumatoid arthritis — clinical benefit occurs within 6 weeks of therapy.

Dose
500 mg per day orally, increased by 3 weekly steps to 2 g per day. This incremental regime helps reduce problems with nausea and vomiting.

Monitoring
The manufacturers recommend monthly full blood counts.

Adverse effects
1 Nausea, vomiting, bloating, dyspepsia or diarrhoea in 33% of patients.
2 Headaches, dizziness and malaise in 20%.

6 Therapy

6.1 Drug therapy

3 Mucocutaneous symptoms such as skin rashes, mouth ulcers, hair thinning and hypersensitivity reactions.
4 Blood — macrocytic anaemia. Leukopenia and neutropenia are potentially hazardous complications unrelated to dose, but appear to occur more frequently in patients with rheumatoid arthritis than those with inflammatory bowel disease.
5 Other: reversible reduction in quantity and quality of spermatogenesis. Alveolitis is rare.

Corticosteroids
Corticosteroids have both anti-inflammatory and immunosuppressive effects and may be administered orally, parenterally and by intra-articular injection. The comparative pharmacology of the glucocorticoids is presented in Table 6.3.

Oral preparations

Indications
Rheumatoid arthritis, systemic lupus erythematosus, dermatopolymyositis, vasculitides, polymyalgia rheumatica.

Table 6.3. Comparison of glucocorticoid pharmacology

Duration of action	Potency	Mineralocorticoid activity
Short (24–36 h)		
Hydrocortisone	1	+
Cortisone	4	−
Prednisolone	4	−
Methylprednisolone	5	−
Intermediate (<48 h)		
Triamcinalone	5	−
Long (<48 h)		
Betamethasone	25	−
Dexamethasone	30	−

6 Therapy

6.1 Drug therapy

Doses
Doses should be kept as low as possible. It is normal to use enteric-coated preparations where possible because of the association with gastritis and peptic ulceration. Soluble prednisolone phosphate, well diluted, is helpful in patients with dyspepsia.

Adverse effects
1 Adrenal suppression — patients on long-term corticosteroid treatment should not stop their tablets suddenly, should inform other doctors they are receiving such treatment and should keep a corticosteroid identity card on their person with details of dosage instructions.
2 Corticosteroid-induced Cushing's syndrome. Changes in appearance include obesity, 'mooning' of the face, osteoporosis, skin atrophy and psychiatric symptoms. Late effects include benign intra-cranial hypertension, aseptic necrosis of bone, glaucoma, posterior subcapsular cataract and pancreatitis. Hypertension, hirsuitism, acne, menstrual disturbances and fluid retention are seen in ACTH-induced Cushing's syndrome.

Parenteral therapy
Pulsed intravenous therapy — methylprednisolone may be given as a large intravenous infusion (500 mg — 1 g), which should be given over at least 30 min, as there have been reports of sudden death following rapid administration. Aseptic necrosis of bone, especially of the hips is a hazard.

Hydrocortisone — this is given intravenously as the hemisuccinate in acute adrenal insufficiency and when oral steroids cannot be given (during the perioperative period).

Intra-articular preparations: 20–40 mg of triamcinolone are usually given into large joints, smaller amounts in lesser joints, as in the fingers (see section 7.1).

6 Therapy

6.1 Drug therapy

Immunosupressive therapy

Azathioprine
This is a purine analogue, which is converted in the liver to 6-mercaptopurine. This in turn is oxidized by xanthine oxidase; hence the possible interaction between patients taking azathioprine and allopurinol.

Indications
Rheumatoid arthritis, systemic lupus erythematosus. It is one of the better tolerated of the immunosuppressives and has a lower frequency of side effects. It has been used with success as a corticosteroid-sparing agent in patients with connective tissue diseases requiring unacceptably high doses of corticosteroids. Teratogenesis does not appear to be a problem with azathioprine.

Dose
Up to 2.5 mg/kg/day, with a ceiling dose of 150 mg/day. Start at 50 mg and build up by 25 mg each week to reduce nausea and vomiting.

Monitoring
2-weekly blood counts for a month, then monthly.

Adverse reactions
1 Nausea and vomiting.
2 Neutropenia, pancytopenia and thrombocytopenia are rare.
3 Macrocytosis is common and results from folate antagonism. It is of no importance unless accompanied by anaemia. It can be reversed by stopping the drug and giving additional folic acid.
4 Allergic hepatitis responds to drug withdrawal.
5 Oncogenesis — increased frequency of malignancy, particularly affecting the lymphoid tissues, when larger doses are used. So far this has not been a serious problem in the treatment of rheumatoid arthritis.

6 Therapy

6.1 Drug therapy

6 Sepsis — as with all immunosuppressives, infection can be a problem especially in the elderly and may present atypically. Herpes zoster and cytomegalovirus infections are the most troublesome.

Methotrexate
Methotrexate interferes with dihydrofolate reductase, important in folate synthesis. Its mode of action in the treatment of rheumatic disease is not clear.

Indications
Rheumatoid arthritis, intractable psoriatic arthritis, Reiter's syndrome and polymyositis. A clinical response occurs within 6 weeks.

Dose
Initial dose is 5–7.5 mg orally once a week. The therapeutic dose ranges between 7.5–15 mg/week with a maximum of 20 mg/week. The parenteral route may also be used.

Monitoring
Weekly full blood count for a month, then monthly. Liver function tests every 2 months.

Adverse effects
1 Hepatotoxicity. Minor abnormalities of liver function are common, affecting about 20% of patients. They respond to drug withdrawal or reduction in dosage and are not predictors of the more serious complication, hepatic fibrosis. This latter has been seen especially in patients who take alcohol while on the drug. Patients should be advised to abstain from or restrict alcohol to 80 g/week. The drug is contraindicated in heavy drinkers.
2 GI upset presents mainly as nausea and diarrhoea and may settle spontaneously or ease with reduction in dosage. Mouth ulcers can also occur.
3 Pancytopenia occurs with methotrexate and necessitates

6 Therapy

6.1 Drug therapy

frequent full blood count estimations. These need to be performed weekly on drug introduction and monthly after stabilization.

4 Interstitial pneumonitis has been associated with methotrexate, especially in high dose intravenous therapy. The drug should not be given to patients with pre-existing lung disease.

5 Oligospermia may develop during therapy but is reversible on stopping the drug.

Note that there is no evidence of increased carcinogenesis. Methotrexate is contraindicated in pregnancy.

Liver biopsy is indicated for persistently abnormal enzymes, development of hypoalbuminaemia, and after 2 years or 1500 mg of therapy.

Baseline biopsy is only indicated if there is a history of alcohol abuse, liver disease or morbid obesity. The drug is excreted renally and should be avoided in patients with a creatinine clearance of less than 50–60 ml/min.

Cyclophosphamide
This alkylating agent interferes with DNA replication by cross-linkage via alkyl groups of the DNA molecule. It may be administered orally or intravenously and is activated by hepatic metabolism. Sixty per cent of the drug is excreted renally.

Indications
Severe rheumatoid arthritis, vasculitis, glomerulonephritis with systemic lupus erythematosus. Despite its toxicity, cyclophosphamide will sometimes bring about remission when all else fails.

Dose
Orally up to 2 mg/kg/day; doses of 50 or 70 mg a day may be effective. It may also be given as i.v. boluses of 750–1000 mg/m^2,

6 Therapy

6.1 Drug therapy

covered by 500 mg−1 g of methyl prednisolone.
Adequate hydration is essential whilst taking the drug.

Monitoring
Blood count 2-weekly for the first month, then monthly.

Adverse effects
1 Abdominal pain, nausea, vomiting, and rarely diarrhoea.
2 Alopecia (rare if dose is built up gradually).
3 Marrow suppression.
4 Infertility — failure of sperm motility and amenorrhoea.
5 Haemorragic cystitis which may proceed to bladder fibrosis and carcinoma. The cystitis occurs at any time, its frequency being reduced by maintaining a dilute urine at all times.
6 Oncogenesis, especially lymphomas and leukaemias.
7 Others: hypogammaglobulinaemia, pulmonary fibrosis.

Chlorambucil
This is an orally administered immunosuppressive agent which has less toxicity than cyclophosphamide, but is less efficacious.

Indications
Severe rheumatoid arthritis.

Monitoring
2-weekly full blood count for the first month, then monthly.

Adverse reactions
1 Marrow suppression especially neutropenia or thrombocytopenia.
2 Others: gastrointestinal upset, hepatotoxicity, oncogenesis, infertility.

6 Therapy

6.2 Rehabilitation

6.2 Rehabilitation

Current therapies are limited in their impact on the patient with musculoskeletal disorders and patients with chronic rheumatic disease face many problems at home, socially and at work. Rehabilitation involves both physiotherapy and occupational therapy as well as the medical social worker. Close liaison with the medical and nursing staff is essential.

The physiotherapist

The physiotherapist's role in the treatment of rheumatic diseases is one of assessment, rehabilitation and education.

Assessment

When a patient first attends the physiotherapy department a careful and detailed assessment is taken to:
- Determine the best methods of treatment for that patient.
- Provide information for the other members of the team.
- Give baseline information for monitoring therapy.
- Give information to the patient.

The assessment includes subjective and objective measurements of pain, range of movement, muscle strength and muscle wasting, functional abilities and social problems.

Aims of physiotherapy

The aim of physiotheraphy treatment is to:
- Relieve pain.
- Reduce swelling.
- Improve range of movement.
- Improve function and independence.
- Improve posture and gait.
- Prevent or correct deformity.
- Educate the patient.

6 Therapy

6.2 Rehabilitation

Methods of treatment

Relief of pain and swelling. This is necessary before exercise therapy. Prior aspiration and injection of painful joints with corticosteroid where appropriate can be very helpful. The most commonly used forms of pain relieving treatment are:
  moist heat (in the form of hydropacks);
  ice packs;
  ultrasound for localized soft tissue lesions (e.g. supraspinatus tendinitis), although it may be harmful in overtly inflammatory lesions.

Improve range of movement and muscle strength. Exercise therapy can be passive, assisted or resisted, isodynamic or isometric, depending on the effects required. Muscle power and range of movement can be increased by the use of:
  slings;
  springs;
  weights;
  manual resistance.

Hydrotherapy. Has an important role in the treatment of rheumatic diseases. The warmth of the water helps to relieve pain and movement is facilitated by the buoyancy of the water.

Improve function and independence. By improving the patient's strength and range of movement, function should also improve, but close work with the occupational therapist will be required.

Improve gait. A patient's posture and gait may be improved by:
  increasing muscle strength, especially the anti-gravity muscles;
  correcting any leg length discrepancy;
  provision of suitable walking aids and footwear.

Prevent or correct deformity. Initially the patient will adopt a

6 Therapy

6.2 Rehabilitation

posture or position that affords maximum pain relief, i.e. a position that minimizes stretch on swollen joints and surrounding soft tissues.

Subsequent contractures may develop with muscle atrophy and pain-induced muscle spasm. The physiotherapist's approach to the prevention of deformities depends on:

educating the patient;
exercise therapy;
passive stretching of contracted soft tissue;
splinting.

Education. Education and advice to the patient continues throughout their therapy. This involves not only reassurance about the condition but also advice about long-term management. Exercises to perform at home are also taught for strengthening muscles and increasing mobility.

The occupational therapist

The occupational therapist assesses and treats disability. The aim is to help the patient achieve and maintain independence in all 'activities of daily living' (ADL). This applies equally to the newly diagnosed patient as to the seriously disabled.

Assessment

The patient is assessed both by interview and by observation to pinpoint areas of difficulty in aspects of work, home and social life. These include:

independence at work and socially;
washing, personal care, bathing;
dressing, feeding;
mobility, transfers;
cooking, housework;
hobbies, leisure activities, communication.

6 Therapy

6.2 Rehabilitation

Aids to daily living
Advice is given to help resolve problems by use of specific aids and equipment. Patients are instructed on their safe and efficient use.

Joint protection
The aim is to advise the patient how to reduce stress on the affected joints by using certain joints or joint positions in preference to others to minimize pain and avoid further damage. Efficiency in carrying out various tasks is also taught and patients are encouraged to incorporate rest periods when necessary.

Splinting
Resting splints are provided during periods of active disease.
Protective splinting may be used on certain joints such as the elbows.
Corrective splinting is employed to help overcome flexion or deviation deformities.

Home assessment
Patients are assessed at home to discover the practical difficulties related to the home environment and how these can be overcome. These include:
ramps instead of steps;
bath aids;
hand rails to promote stability and avoid falls;
adaptations of kitchen, bathroom, telephone and other equipment.

The medical social worker
Social workers aim to assist patients and their families to find solutions to their social problems. This is achieved through counselling and support as well as giving advice regarding resources.

6 Therapy

6.2 Rehabilitation

Table 6.4. Resources available to help the disabled patient

Social service resources
Meals on wheels
Home care assistants (home helps)
Day centres — for elderly and handicapped people
Residential accommodation
Community social workers

Voluntary organizations
For example:
ACROSS — holidays in Europe for handicapped people
Arthritis Care
Lupus Society
NASS — National Ankylosing Spondylitis Society
RADAR — Royal Association for Disability and Rehabilitation
NOS — National Osteoporosis Society

Counselling and support
Social workers receive training in counselling and family work. They can therefore offer emotional support and guidance to those faced with the effects of a disabling illness and help them to find ways to cope, particularly with the many losses they experience such as health, independence and the status, money and satisfaction gained from being employed.

Advice regarding resources
Social workers acquire a wide knowledge of resources with which they can put their clients in touch (Table 6.4, and Appendix 2). Some social workers specialize in the area of welfare rights, developing a thorough knowledge of the DHSS system and the benefits to which disabled people are entitled (Table 6.5). Social workers familiarize themselves with other systems which their clients often find daunting, such as housing provision.

6 Therapy

6.2 Rehabilitation

Table 6.5. Allowances for the disabled

Attendance allowance (leaflet NI 205)
Paid to individual requiring considerable support due to severe physical or mental disability. A higher rate is payable to people requiring help day and night. The person applying must need for 6 months:
frequent attention for help with bodily functions *or*
constant supervision to avoid substantial danger to the applicant or others by day or by night

Severe disablement allowance (leaflet NI 252)
This benefit is payable to people unable to work because of severe mental or physical disablement. To qualify the applicant has to be aged between 16 and 65 and assessed as at least 80% disabled

Mobility allowance (leaflet NI 211)
Persons are eligible if they are aged between 5 and 65 and are unable or almost unable to walk because of physical disability

Assistance with fares to work (leaflet DPL 13)
This is payable to severely disabled persons who are unable to use public transport to get to work and who incur extra travelling expenses as a result. This leaflet is available from Jobcentres or Employment Offices

Invalid care allowance (leaflet NI 212)
Can be claimed by men or single women of working age who are unable to work because they are caring for a severely disabled relative receiving an attendance allowance (eligibility of married women is under review)

For information on other benefits, such as help with heating bills, see leaflet HB 1 'Help for Handicapped People' or FB 2, 'Which Benefit?'. Leaflets may be obtained by writing to the local Social Security Office or, DHSS Leaflets Unit, PO Box 21, Stanmore, Middlesex HA7 1AY

6.3 Surgery

Preparation

General measures
A recent chest X-ray, haemoglobin, white count and biochemical profile, in addition to a general clinical check-up and blood pressure measurements are required.

Specific measures
- X-rays of the part to be operated on in two views. Always get X-rays of the opposite part in the surgery of paired limb joints.
- In patients with rheumatoid arthritis or ankylosing spondylitis, ask for a lateral view of the neck in flexion to exclude cervical subluxation.
- Consider preoperative transfusion if the haemoglobin level is 10 g/dl or less.
- Give 100 mg hydrocortisone hemisuccinate solution intravenously with the premedication and another 100 mg on leaving the operating room for patients on long-term corticosteroid therapy. Repeat postoperatively if vomiting precludes oral treatment.

Specific joints

Wrists and hands
The chief indications for hand surgery in rheumatoid arthritis are restoration of function. The chief cause of loss of function is tendon damage, for example adhesion or nodules in the flexor sheaths blocking active flexion, rupture of extensor tendons with finger drop, displacement of tendon lines of force, causing ulnar deviation.

The following operations are usually helpful:
repair of ruptured tendons;
carpal tunnel decompression;

6 Therapy

6.3 Surgery

    stabilization of flail hyperextended thumbs;
    arthrodeses of subluxed radiocarpal joints;
    removal of the lower end of ulna for dorsal subluxation of the ulnar blocking supination or extension at the wrist.
Generally of less functional benefit are:
    replacement arthroplasties of metacarpophalangeal and interphalangeal joints;
    removal of trapezium in thumb base osteoarthritis;
    attempts at early synovectomy in rheumatoid arthritis.
Special precautions must be taken if there are signs of a complicating arteritis. A preliminary brachial angiogram under the anaesthetic may be needed.

Elbows

Successful procedures include:
    removal of the radial head if displaced;
    removal of antecubital synovial cysts if blocking movement or compromising the interosseous nerve;
    joint replacement arthroplasty in severe disease.

Shoulder

- Replacement arthroplasties relieve pain but seldom increase range of movement, probably because of concurrent muscle wasting.
- Excision arthroplasty of the acromioclavicular joint is sometimes needed.

Neck

Atlanto-axial subluxation may occur quite early in rheumatoid arthritis and in late ankylosing spondylitis. Subluxations at lower levels in rheumatoid arthritis are potentially more serious as there is less room for the spinal cord. Subluxations of the neck are not operated on unless:
    there is considerable pain;
    there are signs of pressure on nerve roots or cord.

6 Therapy

6.3 Surgery

Operations usually involve bone grafts and internal splinting. For severe lower cervical subluxations, halo or minerva splints may be needed.

In ankylosing spondylitis with gross flexion of an ankylosed neck, such that the sufferer cannot look forwards when walking, cervical osteotomy may be done. There are special problems in intubation and anaesthetization and the patient will return from the theatre in a halo splint, which has to be worn until the neck has fused in the corrected position.

Spine
Rheumatology patients may need spinal operations in the following conditions:
  decompression for spinal stenosis due to prolapsed disc, Paget's disease or spondylolisthesis;
  osteotomy for flexed lumbar spine in ankylosing spondylitis;
  fusion of secondary fractures in late ankylosing spondylitis;
  operations for prolapsed disc.

Hips
Replacement arthroplasty is now the most common operation. Indications for joint replacement include:
1 Severe pain, especially if interfering with patient's sleep.
2 Loss of essential mobility.
3 Otherwise good functional capacity.
4 Loss of stability (Trendelenburg sign).
5 Radiographic evidence of destruction.

Four out of the above five are usually required, but operation may also depend on the intensity of any one of the above, on the natural history and needs of the patient. Age is not necessarily a factor, but young people in their thirties remain the poorest prognostic group. The cumulative failure rate is about 13% at 10 years.

Complications of the operation include:
loosening (about 6%);

6 Therapy

6.3 Surgery

early infection 2%;
heterotropic ossification, which restricts range of motion;
nerve compression 0.7%;
unequal leg length.

Postoperative rehabilitation involves:
avoidance of adduction, rotation and flexion greater than 90°;
partial weight bearing begins on second or third day with cemented prostheses;
partial weight bearing for 6 weeks in porous coated hips (to allow for bony ingrowth);
range of motion exercises should be in the anatomic plane.

Low-dose anticoagulants reduce the incidence of post-operative thrombo-embolism and are given from 24 h after operation for up to 6 weeks.

Osteotomy may be used instead of joint replacement in the younger age group.

Knees

Osteotomy is performed for varus, valgus or flexion deformities. These are usually splinted internally and the patient's legs are kept in plaster of Paris until union has begun, when gentle exercises may be started.

Joint replacements are of two types:
constrained; used for knees with unstable ligaments in advanced rheumatoid arthritis where the patient is not expected to do much walking because of the condition of the other joints;
unconstrained; mimic the natural freedom of movement, allowing flexion only when the knee is in extension, but permitting flexion and rotation when the knee is bent.

Indications include:
severe pain;
loss of function;
varus deformity of 20–35°.

Complications are similar to those with hip replacement.

6 Therapy

6.3 Surgery

Failure rates are higher than hip replacement and depend on the prosthesis used, being greatest with the full constrained hinge. Postoperative low dose anticoagulation is given as with hip replacement.

Postoperative rehabilitation depends to some extent on type of prosthesis used:
 constant passive motion postoperatively;
 partial weight bearing followed by transition to crutch weight bearing;
 limit flexion to 90°;
 avoid kneeling or twisting the knee with cemented prostheses.

Ankles and feet
Ankle arthroplasty provides pain relief, but not much extra movement. Triple arthrodesis (talus, calcaneum, navicular) can be used for destruction of subtaloid and posterior tarsal joints.

For distorted toes, operations range from simple balancing osteotomies, done as a day case, on one or more toes to allow prominent metatarsal heads to find their own level with the others, through to complicated excision and reconstruction arthroplasties of the Kates–Kessel type (in which the metatarsal heads are removed along a shallow arc and the toes are replaced using Kirschner wires to hold them postoperatively).

It is important to make sure that the circulation in the feet is adequate preoperatively. A history of arteritis or neuropathy should exclude the patient from operation unless a femoral angiogram or other study discloses good circulation, including to the toes.

Biopsies

Elbow nodules
These must be removed through a longitudinal incision otherwise the skin tends to gape on flexion of the elbow. For

orientation it is best to remove a small ellipse of skin with the nodule.

Rectal biopsies
These are done through a sigmoidoscope when arteritis or amyloidosis is suspected.

Muscle biopsies
These are commonly taken from the deltoid or the vastus lateralis. The sample should be taken along the line of the muscle, then positioned on a piece of cardboard and allowed slightly to air dry before being fixed, otherwise it will curl up making orientation difficult. Special fixatives may be needed. Check with the pathology department first. Avoid muscles that have been used for EMG studies.

Temporal artery biopsy
A vertical incision is made about 3 cm above and anterior to the tragus, the artery is tied at both ends and a section excised. It should be air dried on card before being fixed.

Synovial biopsy
This can be done at arthroscopy or by means of a special biopsy needle inserted into the supra patella pouch. The needle has a cutting side opening and a central cutting trocar which removes material pushed into the side opening of the needle.

Skin biopsy
This may be needed in systemic lupus for flourescent studies, or for diagnosis of drug-associated rashes, psoriasis, etc. A punch biopsy is often adequate. Wherever possible biopsy affected skin. If immunofluorescence is required, the biopsy should be divided in two, half placed on cardboard and fixed, the other put in a container on a piece of gauze and taken to the laboratory. This should be arranged with the pathologist beforehand.

6 Therapy

6.4 Chiropody and shoe prescription

6.4 Chiropody and shoe prescription

Arthritic conditions such as rheumatoid arthritis can cause severe foot problems, because of inflammation and the deformities that may result. The provision of suitable footwear may do much to decrease pain and increase mobility in these patients.

The following points should be considered when prescribing footwear for an arthritic patient.

- Crippled fingers may not be able to do up laces.
- With unequal leg length secondary strains will be put on the lumbar spine and on the knee of the longer limb unless compensated for by raised heels.
- A patient with flexed knees will need higher heels unless there is sufficient dorsiflexion in the ankle to compensate. Similar considerations apply to varus and valgus deformities of the knees.
- A patient with stiff ankles will not be able to point his toes in order to get the foot into a shoe with a normal opening. Extending lacing right down to the toes will be necessary.
- Watch for oedema; lacing is the only satisfactory method of closing a shoe which can accommodate variable foot volume.
- Look out for arteritis and neuropathy with accompanying sensory changes; such patients experience paraesthesiae and no shoe will ever feel as though it fits.
- In diabetic arthropathy skin sensibility may be so diminished that a damaging, ill-fitting shoe may be accepted as comfortable.
- Patients with inadequate circulation or with systemic sclerosis may need the additional insulation provided by a fur-lined shoe or boot.

Insocks

This is the technical name for what are usually called insoles. Insocks should be avoided if possible. It is better to prescribe a shoe with the desired sole contour built in.

6 Therapy

6.4 Chiropody and shoe prescription

Shoes
There are three types of shoe available:
 traditional bespoke shoes:
 shoes made to plaster of Paris casts;
 'depth' shoes.

Traditional bespoke shoes. These are the smartest shoes, the most expensive and have the longest delivery time.

Shoes made to plaster of Paris casts. Casts of the foot are taken and sent away to a central manufacturer. The product is a very light shoe (important for patients with crippled legs). Delivery time is less than with bespoke shoes and the cost is a third to a half that of a traditional shoe.

'Depth' shoes. These are 'off the shelf' shoes held in a central store. A wide choice of lengths and widths is available and extra depth is built into the shoe to allow the insertion of an individually contoured insock. The method is suitable with less severe deformities and is much cheaper.

Other footwear. Felt boots can be provided for very crippled people who are unlikely to do much walking because of problems elsewhere.
 Footwear made of foam plastic or nylon felt can be provided for inpatients through the hospital supplies department. These can be modified by adding or removing foam liners or by cutting holes to accommodate bony prominences or protruding toes. They are useful for patients undergoing rehabilitation for other limb joints. They are also useful for patients with ulcerated feet as they can be easily cleaned and sterilized.

Modifications to shoes. The method of closure can be by laces, by a leather bar across the upper part of the foot, by a return velcro strap, or by zip and ring. Lacing can be extended to toe

6 Therapy

6.4 Chiropody and shoe prescription

level. For patients with difficult feet due to protruding toes, sandals may be the only practical choice.

Heel height. This will normally be about 1 cm greater than the sole height. Elderly women who have always worn a shoe with a higher heel may need 2–3 cm otherwise they may feel unstable.

Precise adjustment of heel height is necessary for people with stiff ankles; a little too much or too little will lead to pain.

Difference in leg length of more than 1 cm cannot be compensated simply by heel additions — some will also be needed to be wedged off into the sole.

Floating in and floating out. These describe extension of the heel towards or away from the midline to help counteract a tendency for the patient to turn the foot in the shoe over to one side. Floats of more than 0.5 cm are seldom required.

Wedged heels. Heels can be wedged to make them higher on one side or the other to help counteract valgus or varus deformity. The sole must also be wedged in a similar amount.

Extended heels. The heel is extended forward to the sole and provides additional strength in the middle of the shoe.

Adaptions for special purposes
- Oil-proof materials used for people working in oily surroundings (lathe operators, petrol pump attendants, etc.)
- Avoid microcellular rubber soling for those who work where metal swarf is a hazard — it is picked up by the material and works through to the foot.
- It is difficult to waterproof prescription shoes — it is better for the patient to wear a rubber overboot (farmers, outdoor workers).

6 Therapy

6.4 Chiropody and shoe prescription

Attachments of braces
For the common valgus deformity at the ankle, it is better in mild disease to prescribe a boot rather than a shoe, and with more severe disease to attach a below knee brace, described as 'outside iron with inside T-strap'.

Difficult fitting problems
For seriously protruding toes, it is better to seek a surgical solution — either amputation or osteotomy. No shoe other than a sandal can be expected not to chafe.

Toe tip callosities are a problem in patients whose toes are clawed sufficiently for the tip of the toe to take the weight in walking. A painful callosity forms under the nail, which can be relieved by strapping a roll of dentist's felt underneath the toes, or by the chiropodist fitting a little moulded splint which will push the toe forward.

Prominent bunions and pressure points. A U-shaped adhesive felt pad should be used so that the shoe pressure falls not on the protrusion, but on the ring.

Hallux rigidus. This is a painful condition where the first metatarsophalangeal joint is rigid and cannot properly dorsiflex. The simplest solution is to provide a metatarsal bar under the sole of the shoe so that the patient rocks or rolls over the bar rather than dorsiflexes the toe whilst walking.

Painful subluxation of the metatarsal heads. This can be treated with a metatarsal pad inside the shoe.

Painful calcaneal spurs. A thick adhesive felt pad should have a hole cut in it to correspond to the painful spur. Make a cardboard template first, marking the site of tenderness, and cut the felt accordingly, felt side uppermost.

6 Therapy

6.5 Diet in arthritis

The role of diet in arthritis has received much attention from the lay press. This is fuelled by anecdotal reports of dramatic improvement following dietary manipulation or by the results of short-term studies involving small numbers of patients. It may seem attractive to a patient with a disease such as rheumatoid arthritis over which he has little control to try to regain an active role by following various (sometimes expensive) dietary regimens.

Nevertheless, some experimental evidence does exist which suggests that diet may be important in rheumatoid arthritis.

Diet plays a role in gout and possibly in osteoarthritis.

Gout

Gout is a storage disease of sodium biurate, one of three major excretion products of nitrogen metabolism. Urate levels may be increased by various dietary factors such as:
- Intake of purine rich food such as kidney, liver, brain, anchovies and sardines.
- High alcohol intake (especially beer) by reducing urinary urate and increasing adenine nucleotide turnover.
- Obesity: increased uric acid production and decreased renal excretion.
- Lead toxicity 'saturnine gout': reduced renal uric acid clearance.
- High protein intake.

Gout is also associated with hyperlipidaemia.

Dietary advice to patients
- Weight reduction can reduce serum urate levels.
- Avoid binges of alcohol or purine rich foods which may precipitate acute attacks.
- Moderate intake of these foodstuffs at other times.
- Associated hyperlipidaemia should be treated by an appropriate diet.

6 Therapy

6.5 Diet in arthritis

- Reduce high protein intake.

Osteoarthritis
Obesity is associated with osteoarthritis of the knee and the hand, but not of the hip. There is no good evidence that obesity will cause or accelerate osteoarthritis although it may increase symptoms in weight bearing joints particularly the knee and diets for weight reduction will usually reduce OA knee pain.

Rheumatoid arthritis and other inflammatory arthropathies
Many patients with inflammatory diseases such as rheumatoid arthritis have attempted to modify their disease by dietary means. A proportion of patients can identify particular foodstuffs which they feel exacerbate their disease: red meat, dairy produce and wine are common examples. The results of studies may be confused by the immunosuppressant effect of fasting alone. Convincing evidence of efficacy of dietary regimens is lacking, but results of a few clinical studies are now available.

'The Eskimo diet'
This is based on a diet rich in polyunsaturated fatty acids with eicosapentanoic acid (EPA). EPA is a substrate for prostaglandins of the E_3 series which are less active as inflammatory mediators than their E_2 relatives. Modest improvement of some clinical parameters of disease activity has been reported in clinical trials.

'The Dong diet'
This is a diet free from additives, preservatives, fruit, red meat, herbs and dairy products. There is no evidence for overall benefit, but it has been suggested that selected patients may be helped.

6 Therapy

6.5 Diet in arthritis

Dietary additives
Green-lipped mussel extracts could not be distinguished from dried fish meal in controlled clinical studies.

Feverfew (tanacetum) has shown effects on platelets and polymorphs in *in vitro* studies, although no clinical studies are available.

Dietary advice to patients
- A patient with widespread inflammatory arthropathy often requires a high protein, high carbohydrate diet to compensate for increased tissue catabolism.
- Patients should be advised against following faddish expensive diets of doubtful value.
- You will probably be asked about 'acids' in the diet. Explain that the only rheumatic disease connected with an acid is gout. All the other dietary acids (citric, malic, lactic, acetic, tartaric, ascorbic, nicotinic) are foods or vitamins.

Investigation of a patient for food intolerance
If a patient is convinced that symptoms are related to foodstuffs then several options are available to investigate the possibility.

Dietary manipulation
- A patient with constant symptoms attributed to milk should improve after 6 days on mineral water alone (longer in an older subject).
- An alternative is a hypoallergenic diet (e.g. white fish and pears).
- Medication may have to be stopped (most tablets contain corn starch).
- The suspected items should then be reintroduced one at a time and a diary kept of symptoms. Foods associated with any adverse symptoms should be excluded.

6   Therapy

6.5   Diet in arthritis

Radioallergosorbent test
The radioallergosorbent test (RAST) measures allergen-specific IgE antibodies. However, it is non-specific, expensive and limited in application to certain foods.

7 Skills in rheumatology

7.1 Joint aspiration and injection, 279

7.2 Arthroscopy and bone biopsy, 293

7 Skills in rheumatology

7.1 Joint aspiration and injection

7.1 Joint aspiration and injection

Benefits of injection
Local injection therapy with corticosteroids has brought about a minor revolution in the treatment of patients with rheumatoid arthritis and similar diseases. There is less need for hospitalization, less need for splinting techniques and physiotherapy to restore muscle strength and the ease, speed and range of joint motion can be regained earlier.

Pain relief is such that many patients with, for example, subacromial bursitis, can be kept at work, where previously they might have had to stay away.

Complications
- Infection.
- Pain may be increased especially in the first 24 h following the injection of a tennis elbow, or in calcific periarthritis if the crystalline deposit is disturbed.
- Facial flushing up to 24 h following the injection.
- Skin atrophy at site of injection.
- Tendon rupture if intratendinous injection is inadvertently given.
- Loss of diabetic control especially in 'brittle' diabetics.

General technique
The aspiration and injection of joints is a very safe procedure given a meticulous no-touch technique. Points to follow are:
1 Use disposable needles and syringes and single dose ampoules wherever possible.
2 Hands should be washed and well dried; gloves and masks are not necessary. However, do not talk over an exposed needle.
3 Find the spot where injection is to take place by careful palpation and mark it as a cross with a ball point pen. Disinfect the skin with an isopropyl alcohol swab wiping away the centre

7 Skills in rheumatology

7.1 Joint aspiration and injection

of the cross. The remaining arms of the cross will point to the site of injection.

4 Use a refrigerant spray to anaesthetize the site of injection. It is usually unnecessary to do a preliminary anaesthetization of the capsule of the joint if the technique of injection is good.

5 Always attempt aspiration of fluid first and if successful send the fluid for culture. Fluids that are very thick, greenish or bad smelling are infected. If in doubt do not inject, but wait for the results of microscopy and culture.

6 Be very sure of the diagnosis. For example, an ununited scaphoid fracture may simulate arthritis of the wrist. Check with an X-ray first. This also helps with planning an injection.

7 In a large joint use an adequate bolus by mixing locally-active corticosteroid with 1% lignocaine. Particularly in the knee, an injection of corticosteroid tends to aggregate and stay in one place unless well diluted.

Triamcinolone hexacetonide has proved to be a very satisfactory preparation for local injection into joints. Duration of action is prolonged and there is little, if any, tendency to secondary crystal synovitis. The suggested amounts given in Table 7.1 are worked out in terms of this material and 1% lignocaine.

Which patients?

Joints. Patients with chronic inflammatory diseases (rheumatoid arthritis, psoriatic arthritis, reactive arthritis) are suitable for injection.

In some patients with pyrophosphate arthropathy and persistent effusions, injections of corticosteroids can suppress fluid formation and keep the patient more comfortable. With the exception of the first carpometacarpal joint at the thumb base, osteoarthritic joints usually only gain transient relief following injection.

Table 7.1 Suggested amounts of triamcinolone hexacetonide and lignocaine

Joint	Triamcinolone hexacetonide (mg)	1% Lignocaine (ml)	Notes
Knees	20–40	10	Aspirate large effusions first to reduce tension
Ankles, elbows, subacromial bursa	5–10	5	
Wrists	5	3	
Small joints of hands and feet, temporomandibular, acromioclavicular, sternoclavicular joints	5	2	Use the volume of this mixture that the joint will accept
Soft tissue lesions, bursitis, etc.	5	10	Infiltrate this mixture widely in painful lesions around the trochanters and low back attempting to numb the tender areas

7 Skills in rheumatology

7.1 Joint aspiration and injection

Soft tissues. Inflammatory bursitis, tenosynovitis and enthesitis often respond well to injection.

The patient. The patient should be relaxed. Tense muscles increase the pressure in joints and may make injection impossible.
- Ankles, knees and hips: the patient should be lying supine with the head comfortably supported on pillows.
- Small joints of the fingers, thumbs and wrist: the injection is best done across a desk or table.
- Elbows, shoulders, subacromial spaces and temporomandibular joints: patient should be sitting on the edge of a couch.

How often?
Worries about the possible damage caused by frequent intra-articular corticosteroids are fewer than they used to be. The evidence is that unsuppressed inflammation is more damaging than possible adverse effects of a local corticosteroid.

A good general rule is not to inject the same joint more frequently than every 4 months without considering a change in other therapy (e.g. second-line agent in RA).

The knee joint is most likely to require reinjection. The method gives relief for much longer in other joints, particularly in the small joints of the fingers and toes.

Failure to respond
1 The injection may not have penetrated the joint space. It is a good idea, when learning techniques, to put a small amount of contrast medium in the injection bolus and X-ray afterwards to see where the injection has gone.
2 The main cause of pain in the joint was not arthritis, but the secondary deformities. For example, in a valgus knee, pain may be arising mainly from compression fracture of the lateral tibial

7 Skills in rheumatology

7.1 Joint aspiration and injection

table rather than from the arthritis which damaged the joint in the first place.

Individual joints

Wrists
Wrists are injected in the T-shaped space formed by the radiocarpal and scaphoid-lunate joints (Fig. 7.1). Injections are made with the needle pointed towards the shoulder to correspond to the curve of the radiocarpal joint.

The lower radioulnar joint is most easily found by injecting the dorsal aspect with the needle pointing towards the hand into the space between the lower end of the radius and ulna, until it reaches through into the joint.

Small joints of the hands
Metacarpophalangeal and proximal interphalangeal joints are

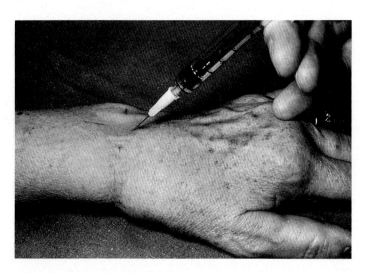

Fig. 7.1 Injection of the wrist.

7   Skills in rheumatology

7.1   Joint aspiration and injection

injected from the side with the tip of the needle coming to lie underneath the extensor expansion.

Palpation finds the joint space but remember that the joint line in the MCP joints is approximately 1 cm distal to the knuckle and that of PIP joints 0.5 cm distal to the knuckle in the lightly flexed fist.

The examiner's finger on the other side of the joint can feel when the joint has been inflated with the injection bolus.

The thumb base joint can be a very successful injection in someone with symptomatic OA at that site (Fig. 7.2).

Elbow

The elbow is injected from the rear. Palpate about 3 cm above the point of the elbow, the depression between the two parts of the triceps tendon. The injection is then made into the olecranon fossa at the appropriate depth.

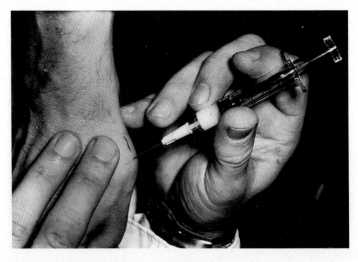

Fig. 7.2 Injection of the 1st carpometacarpal joint in a patient with OA.

7 Skills in rheumatology

7.1 Joint aspiration and injection

Alternatively, the radial head can be located by twisting the forearm whilst palpating the elbow and an injection made just proximal to it in the joint space (Fig. 7.3).

Shoulder
The glenohumeral joint is not always easy to enter. Study an X-ray first. There are two common methods.
1 Anterior, in the space between the head of the humerus and the coracoid process (Fig. 7.4).
2 Posterior (this is easier). The joint line can be approximately palpated and the injection made towards the coracoid process on the other side.

Subacromial bursa
This is best approached from the rear since the space between the head of the humerus and the acromioclavicular arch can most easily be palpated there, particularly in muscular subjects. The injection is made slightly upwards under the acromial arch into a space where injection is easy.

Acromioclavicular joints
These are best injected from in front, the depth of the exploring needle showing when the joint has been located. The joint is of very small capacity.

Sternoclavicular joint and sternomanubrial joint
With careful palpation these can be located and injected.

Temporomandibular joint
This can usually be located by palpation fairly easily and the location is confirmed by asking the patient to open the mouth when the condyle of the mandible will be felt to move forwards.

Hip
Techniques for aspiration and injection of the acetabular joint are

7 Skills in rheumatology

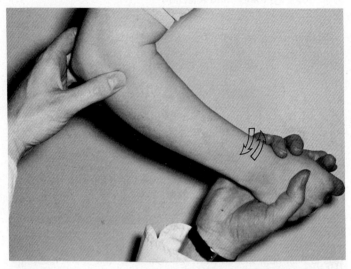

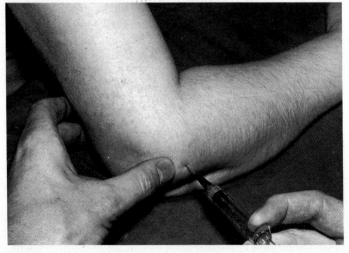

Fig. 7.3 (a) Supination and pronation of the patient's forearm helps to identify the radial head. (b) The injection is made proximal to this.

7 Skills in rheumatology

7.1 Joint aspiration and injection

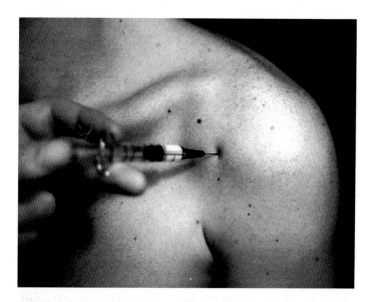

Fig. 7.4 The anterior approach to the shoulder joint is the space between the head of the humerus and the coracoid process.

not easy and appropriate detailed books should be consulted. The most common way is to locate the prominence of the greater trochanter between finger and thumb and mark a point midway between. This corresponds to the base of the neck of the femur. The needle is inserted anterior to this point and redirected parallel to the neck of the femur as indicated on an A–P X-ray of the pelvis. It is gradually redirected closer to the bone until the capsule of the joint is successfully penetrated.

Knee

This is usually considered the easiest joint to enter. It is such a large joint that it can be approached from many different aspects.

7 Skills in rheumatology

7.1 Joint aspiration and injection

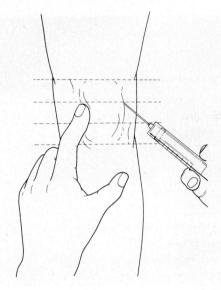

Fig. 7.5 Diagram to show the technique for knee injection using the lateral approach.

The authors favour the lateral approach with the patient lying supine (Fig. 7.5).
1 Subdivide the patella into three horizontal segments.
2 At the junction of middle and upper thirds palpate for the patellofemoral joint line, at the same time pushing the patella laterally to tighten the capsule.
3 Insert the needle along the joint line under the patella towards the suprapatellar pouch, remembering that the joint cavity is only 2 cm beneath the skin.

Ankle
This is best approached from the front. Lateral X-ray should be consulted for the general anatomy.

7 Skills in rheumatology

7.1 Joint aspiration and injection

With the patient supine and the foot slightly plantar flexed, palpate the tendon of the tibialis anterior muscle.

The needle enters the joint tangentially to the articular surface of the talus lateral to the tibialis anterior tendon.

Note that the talotibial (ankle) joint frequently communicates with the posterior subtaloid joint and with the peroneal and posterior tibial groups of tendon sheaths around the ankles.

Intertarsal joints
These are not easy to inject, particularly in fat or oedematous feet.

Small joints
Considerable benefit can be obtained by injecting the intermetatarsal bursae which lie between the heads of the tarsal bones. It is also reasonably easy to inject the metatarsophalangeal joints and with some difficulty, the interphalangeal joints of the toes.

Tendon sheaths, bursae
Benefit can often be obtained by injecting inflamed tendon sheaths or bursae.

Trigger finger may be treated by injecting the appropriate tendon sheath.
1 The needle should be advanced until the tendon is reached.
2 This spot may be recognized by the tendon scratching the end of the needle as the finger is flexed.
3 The end of the needle should be withdrawn slightly and the injection given. The fluid may be seen to run distally along the tendon sheath (Fig. 7.6).

Carpal tunnel may be treated by injecting just on the ulnar side of the palmaris tendon, near or just proximal to the crease at the

7   Skills in rheumatology

7.1   Joint aspiration and injection

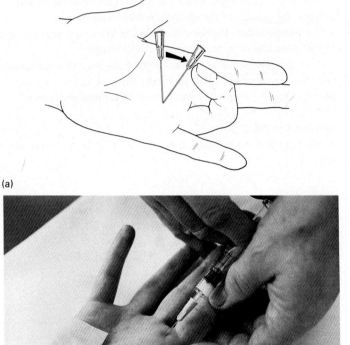

(a)

(b)

Fig. 7.6 (a) The flexor tendon sheath can be identified by a scratching sensation under the needle with flexion of the finger. (b) The needle is then withdrawn slightly and angled to run between the tendon sheath and tendon.

7 Skills in rheumatology

7.1 Joint aspiration and injection

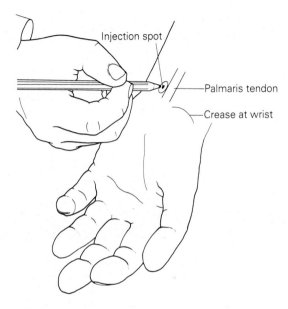

Fig. 7.7 Injection of the carpal tunnel: marking the injection spot.

wrist. The deep fascia is penetrated and a space found into which the injection mixture will run without undue pressure (Fig. 7.7).

Painful enthesitis
The enthesis is the site of the attachment of a muscle or tendon to the bone. It is rich in nerve endings and may become spontaneously painful.
  Common examples include:
  tennis and golfer's elbow (Fig. 7.8);
  attachment of medial ligament of knee to the medial meniscus;
  attachment of long plantar ligament to the calcaneum.
  The principle of injection here is rather different. The fluid to be injected must be injected under pressure. Care must be taken to ensure that the needle is firmly on the syringe.

7 Skills in rheumatology

7.1 Joint aspiration and injection

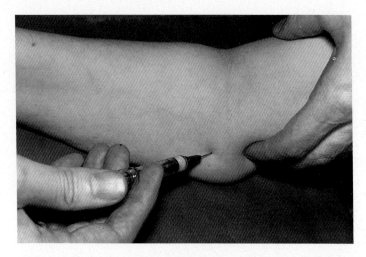

Fig. 7.8 Injection of the insertion of the common flexor tendons in golfer's elbow. The nearby ulnar nerve should be identified and avoided.

Up to 5 ml can be injected in and around the insertion of the wrist extensors to the lateral epicondyle in tennis elbow, up to 2 ml in the region of the medial epicondyle in golfer's elbow (Fig. 7.8). Smaller amounts will be needed elsewhere.

7 Skills in rheumatology

7.2 Arthroscopy and bone biopsy

Arthroscopy

Arthroscopy is the visualization of the cavity of a joint with an endoscope. The arthroscope is a rigid quartz glass rod with an air lens. It is connected to a light source and an eyepiece and there are facilities for connecting it to a still camera or videorecorder.

Knee arthroscopy
Indications include:
- Visual diagnosis.
- Biopsies — culture may be the only way to diagnose tuberculosis and infection with other unusual organisms.
- Inspection of the articular cartilage and meniscal cartilages.
- Operative removal of torn or fissured menisci.

Arthroscopy is now an established technique in the orthopaedic management of meniscal disorders of the knee.

In rheumatology, it is useful for teaching and biopsy work, particularly in relation to chondrocalcinosis and villonodular synovitis.

In rheumatoid arthritis and osteoarthritis, the visual appearances usually give more help than the microscopic ones. The procedure is as follows.
- The patient is sedated with benzodiazepine and is positioned supine on an operating table with the knee slightly flexed.
- Full sterile precautions are taken.
- Local anaesthetic is infiltrated around the site of entry for the arthroscope.
- A trocar and cannula is introduced into the knee to enable the joint fluid and debris to be washed out and replaced by sterile saline from a drip bottle.
- The arthroscope is introduced via a cannula into the knee joint after a small incision has been made in the angle between the patella and patellar tendon on the lateral aspect of the knee.
- The knee is examined systematically starting with the

suprapatellar pouch. It may be necessary to flex the knee to view the medial meniscus.
- Biopsy forceps may be introduced to permit synovial biopsies under direct vision.
- The trocars are removed and the incisions stitched.
- The knee is bandaged and the patient is kept in bed overnight.

The incidental saline lavage of the knee, done as a preliminary to arthroscopy, often seems to be followed by temporary improvement in pain in rheumatoid arthritis. Often an injection of corticosteroid is given into the joint cavity before the incision is closed.

Arthroscopy of the shoulder and hip have been attempted, but have not proved practical for routine work.

Bone biopsy

Indications
Diagnostic:
  osteoporosis;
  osteomalacia;
  Paget's disease;
  secondary deposits in bone, myelomatosis;
  hyperparathyroidism and other metabolic bone diseases.
Monitoring: repeat biopsies to follow effects of treatment.

Preparation of patient
X-ray or isotope bone scan of ilium. Tetracycline double labelling gives more information:
  days 1–3 oxytetracycline 250 mg 3 times a day;
  days 4–14 no tetracycline;
  days 15–17 oxytetracycline 250 mg 3 times a day;
  day 20 biopsy.

7 Skills in rheumatology

7.2 Arthroscopy and bone biopsy

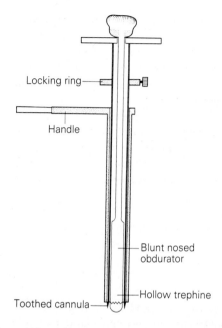

Fig. 7.9 'Stanmore' bone biopsy assembly (after Woolf & Dixon 1988).

Premedication
Diazapam 5–10 mg i.v.

Technique
1 Full aseptic precautions are taken. The patient is supine on the operating table and a small incision 4 cm posterior and inferior to anterosuperior iliac spine is made.
2 Use lignocaine 1% and adrenaline 1 in 200 000 to anaesthetize skin and down to periosteum. Carry out a blunt dissection down to the bone.
3 Introduce the bone biopsy assembly (see Fig. 7.9) with blunt obdurator in place and engage toothed cannula into bone.

7 Skills in rheumatology

7.2 Arthroscopy and bone biopsy

4 Remove obdurator and rotate toothed trephine through outer and inner cortex making sure the stop ring is firmly locked to prevent excessive penetration into iliacus muscle.
5 Keeping the cannula in place, remove trephine which should contain the bone core. If not, replace and cut a little further to loosen the sample.

Note the ease with which the bone can be cut. This varies from rock hard in a normal man to an almost imperceptable resistance to the trephine in an elderly osteoporotic woman.

Close the skin wound with stitch or adhesive strip and apply pressure dressing. Most patients can go home in 2–3 h.

The specimen
This is expelled from the trephine using the blunt obdurator and fixed according to the histologist's instructions. If in doubt use 70% ethanol.

Histomorphometry
After fixation, sectioning and staining the use of fluorescent and ordinary light microscopy permits a large number of measurements to be made, giving information which includes the rates of bone accretion and resorption, osteoblastic and osteoclastic activity and the presence and degree of osteomalacia or other bone disease.

Appendices

1 Useful addresses and information, 299
2 Further reading, 308

Appendices

1 Useful addresses and information

1 Useful addresses and information

Organizations and publications concerned with rheumatic diseases and disability

Organizations fostering research and education
Arthritis and Rheumatism Council for Research (ARC), 41 Eagle Street, London WCIR 4AR. Tel: 01–405 8572.
Funds all kinds of research and education in the field of rheumatic diseases.

National Ankylosing Spondylitis Society (NASS), 6 Grosvenor Crescent, London SW1X 7ER. Tel: 01–235 9585.
Welfare, self-help, education and research into the social consequences of ankylosing spondylitis.

National Osteoporosis Society, Barton Meade House, PO Box 10, Haydon, Radstock, Nr Bath, Avon BA3 3YB. Tel: Radstock 32472.
Education and research into the prevention/treatment of osteoporosis.

Back Pain Association Ltd, Grundy House, Somerset Road, Teddington, Middlesex TW11 8TD. Tel: 01–977 5474.
Funds education and research into the causes and treatment of back pain.

British League Against Rheumatism (BLAR), 41 Eagle Street, London WC1R 4AR. Tel: 01–405 8572.
A federation of all professional and lay organizations in this field. Represents the interests of British rheumatism and arthritis sufferers with regard to national and international governmental agencies and publishes a newsletter and directory of courses and conferences.

Aids and equipment
Biological Engineering Society, Handicap Advisory and Rehabilitation Group, c/o Keith Copeland, Dept. of Biophysics, University College, Gower Street, London WC1. Tel: 01–387 7050 Ext. 288.
Specialist advice, unusual equipment.

Disabled Living Centre, 260 Broad Street, Birmingham 1 B1 2HF. Tel: 021–643 0980.
Exhibition of aids and equipment.

Appendices

1 Useful addresses and information

Disabled Living Foundation, 380–384 Harrow Road, London W.
  Tel: 01–289 6111.
  Provides a comprehensive display of aids and equipment that can be tried. It also provides an excellent information centre.

Egerton Hospital Equipment Ltd, Tower Hill, Horsham, Surrey RH13 7JT.
  Tel: Horsham 3800.
  Makers of electric and other turning beds.

GU Manufacturing Co. Ltd, 28a Devonshire Street, London W1.
  Suppliers of rubber urinals — colloquially known as 'kippers'.

H & C Lifts, 159 St John Street, London EC1V 4JQ.
  Makers of domestic lifts.

Interlock Systems for the Disabled, The Spastics Society,
  Sherrards Industrial Centre, Digswell Hill, Old Welwyn,
  Hertfordshire. Tel: 01–636 5020.
  Produce many simple electrical and electronic aids at reasonable prices.

Maling Rehabilitation Systems Ltd, St Andrew's Way, Industrial
  Estate, Bicester Road, Aylesbury, Buckinghamshire. Tel:
  Aylesbury 86521.
  Electronic environmental control systems advisory service.

Merseyside Aids Centre, Youens Way, East Prescot Road, Liverpool
  L14 2EP.
  Exhibition of aids and equipment.

Newcastle Aids Centre, The Dene Centre, Castle Farm Road, Newcastle
  Upon Tyne NE3 1PH. Tel: 091–284 0480.
  Exhibition of aids and equipment.

The Royal Association for Disability and Rehabilitation (RADAR),
  25 Mortimer Street, London W1N 8AB. Tel: 01–637 5400.
  Has a travelling exhibition of aids.

Tally Surgical Instruments Ltd, 47 Theobald Street, Borehamwood,
  Hertfordshire. Tel: 01–953 7171.
  Makers of ripple cushions and mattresses.

Terry Personal Lifts, Knutsford, Cheshire WA16 8XJ. Tel: Knutsford 0565–3211.
  Makers of interfloor lifts.

Appendices

1 Useful addresses and information

Vessa Ltd, Queen Mary's Hospital, Roehampton, London SW15.
 Tel: 01–788 4422.
 Makers of wheelchairs.

Vitafoam Ltd, Don Mill, Middleton, Manchester 4.
 Makers of sorbo-rubber packs.

Wessex Medical Equipment Co., The Hundred, Romsey, Hampshire F051 OHA. Tel: 0794–830303.
 Makers of electric hoists, lifts and other medical equipment including beds.

Zimmer Orthopaedic Ltd, Bridgend, Glamorgan, Wales.
 Makers of wheelchairs and other equipment.

Books and publications
Dr Wendy Greengross, *Entitled to Love*, Most explicit book on the sexual aspect of disability. Published by Malaby Press, London, in association with the National Fund for Research into Crippling Diseases, 1 Springfield Road, Horsham, Sussex.
Joanna Johnson, *Working at Home*, Information on home employment. Penguin edition.
AA Guide for the Disabled, Automobile Association Hotel Services Dept, PO Box 52, Basingstoke, Hampshire. General useful information relating to suitable accommodation and travelling.
ABC of Services and Information, Disablement Income Group (*DIG*), 28 Commercial Street, London E1.

Journals and newspapers for rheumatism sufferers
ARC, Journal of the Arthritis and Rheumatism Council, 41 Eagle Street, London WC1R 2AR. Tel: 01–405 8572.
Arthritis News, Publication of the British Rheumatism and Arthritis Association, 6 Grosvenor Crescent, London SW1 7ER. Tel: 01–235 0902.
NASS Newsletter, Publication of the National Ankylosing Spondylitis Society, 6 Grosvenor Crescent, London SW1X 7ER. Tel: 01–235 9585.

For lay readers
Jayson M.I.V. & Dixon A. St J., (1984) *Rheumatism and Arthritis — What You Should Know about the Problems and Treatment*, Pan Books, London SW10 9PG.

Appendices

1 Useful addresses and information

Car conversions and driving advice

Automobile & Industrial Developments Ltd, Queensdale Works, Queensthorpe Road, Sydeham, London SE24 4PJ. Tel: 01-698 3451.
Specialists in conversions for all types of cars.

Brig-Ayd Controls, 1 Margery Lane, Tewin, Welwyn, Hertfordshire AL6 OPJ.
Specialists in all types of conversions.

Cowal Medical Aids Ltd, 32 New Pond Road, Holmer Green, Buckinghamshire HP15 6SU. Tel: Holmer Green 3065.
Specialists in conversions for all vehicles.

DBS Garages (Cranleigh) Ltd, High Street, Cranleigh, Surrey GU6 8AG.
Conversion of Renault 4 high roof car. Has portable ramps.

Feeny & Johnson Ltd, Alperton Lane, Wembley, Middlesex HA0 1JJ. Tel: 01-998 4458/9.
Provide a national and worldwide service. Write to head office for full details of service and controls.

Midland Cylinder Rebores Ltd, Torrington Avenue, Coventry. Tel: Coventry 462422.
Specialists in all types of conversions.

Mini-Van Conversion, Modern Vehicle Construction Ltd, Darwin Close, Commercial Road, Reading, Berkshire.
Has a raised roof, double doors and a portable ramp.

Mini-Van Conversion, Roots Maidstone Ltd, Mill Street, Maidstone, Kent ME15 6YD.
Has raised roof, horse-box type tail gate.

Reselco Invalid Carriages Ltd, 262-264 King Street, Hammersmith, London W6. Tel: 01-748 5053/4.
Specialists in conversions for all types of cars.

Banstead Place Mobility Centre, Park Road, Banstead, Surrey. Tel: 073 73-56222.
Information on car adaptations and will assess individual sufferers' needs.

Appendices

1 Useful addresses and information

Educational opportunities for rheumatism sufferers

The Advisory Centre for Education (ACE), 32 Trumpington Street, Cambridge.
   Advice on all educational matters.

Association for Special Education, 19 Hamilton Road, Wallasey, Cheshire L45 9VE. Tel: 051–522 3451.
   For children.

Council for Accreditation of Correspondence Colleges, 27 Marylebone Road, London NW1. Tel: 01–935 54391.
   Has lists and information relating to courses.

National Institute of Adult Education, 35 Queen Anne Street, London W1.
   Full information on courses and classes through local educational departments.

Open University Degree Courses, Open University, PO Box 48, Bletchley, Buckinghamshire.
   Further degree standard education. A most helpful and progressive body in meeting educational requirements of the disabled.

The Royal Association for Disability and Rehabilitation (RADAR), 25 Mortimer Street, London W1N 8AB. Tel: 01–637 5400.
   Information and advice on education problems.

Employment, legal aid and housing

Carr's Rehabilitation Employment Advisory Service, 48 William IV Street, London WC2. Tel: 01–836 5506.
   A private company that specializes in obtaining employment for disabled people.

Centre of Environment for the Handicapped, 126 Albert Street, Camden, London NW1 7NE. Tel: 01–267 6111.
   Advice and guidance about house design.

Disabled Drivers' Insurance Bureau, 292 Hale Lane, Edgware, Middlesex HA8 8NB. Tel: 01–985 3135.
   Advice about insurance.

Horder Centre for Arthritis, Maurien Dufferin Place, Crowborough, Sussex TN6 1XP.
   Residential care and training.

Appendices

1   Useful addresses and information

The Joint Committee on Mobility for the Disabled, Wanborough Manor, Wanborough, Guildford, Surrey GU3 2JR. Tel: Guildford 810484.
  Advice and information about transport problems.

Legal Aid, New Legal Aid, PO Box 9, Nottingham NG1 6DS.
  Advice and information regarding legal aid.

The National Federation of Housing Associations, 86 Strand, London WC2R 0EG. Tel: 01–836 2741.
  Guide to all housing associations.

Parking privileges
The yellow-brown discs which give parking privileges are obtained on the recommendation of a doctor or hospital. They apply to the car carrying a disabled person, whether driven or passenger. To qualify, an arthritic sufferer must be considered virtually unable to walk. This generally means serious foot, knee or hip disease.

Rates relief
Most physically disabled people are entitled to rates relief, at least on their garage. Apply to the local valuation officer for further details.

Voting
Physically disabled people are entitled to postal voting. Apply to the local electoral registrar for details.

Finance
The Aids Trust, Sutton Waldon, Blanford, Dorset.
  Financial support for the purchase of aids and equipment.

Birmingham Settlement Money Advice Centre, 318 Summer Lane, Birmingham B19 3RL. Tel: 021–359 3562.
  Debt counselling agency.

Citizens' Advice Bureau, 26 Bedford Square, London WC1B 3HU. Tel: 01–636 4066, also local offices.
  Advice on hire purchase mortgages, tax, insurance, etc.

Citizens' Rights Officer, 1 Macklin Street, Drury Lane, London WC2B 5NH.
  Will represent people at tribunals, advise over means test,

Appendices

1 Useful addresses and information

supplementary benefits, all at no cost.

Claimants' Union, The Albany, Creek Road, London SE8. Tel: 01–612 1047.
Self-help groups, assist in benefit claims and appeals.

Disability Alliance, 96 Portland Place, London W1. Tel: 01–794 1536.
Advice and information on social security benefits.

Disablement Incomes Group (DIG), Attlee House, Toynbee Hall, 28 Commercial Street, London E1 6LR.
Pressure group — fights for better economic and social position for all disabled. Advice on social security benefits.

The Royal Association for Disability and Rehabilitation (RADAR), 25 Mortimer Street, London W1N 8AB. Tel: 01–637 5400.
Produce leaflets on such matters as income tax rate rebates.

General welfare
Arthritis Care, 5 Grosvenor Crescent, London W1N 8AB. Tel: 01–235 0902.
The largest national society for welfare of rheumatism sufferers, also has information on travel and holiday homes.

National Ankylosing Spondylitis Society, 5 Grosvenor Crescent, London SW1X 7ER. Tel: 01–235 9585.
For ankylosing spondylitis sufferers.

The Lupus Society, c/o Arthritis Care, 5 Grosvenor Crescent, London SW1X 7ER. Tel: 01–235 0902.
For sufferers from lupus erythematosis.

Scleroderma Society, Pamela Webster, Chairman, 61 Sandpits Lane, St. Albans, Hertfordshire.

Association of Disabled Professionals, c/o Mrs P Marchant, The Stables, 73 Pound Road, Banstead, Surrey SM7 2HU.

British Red Cross Society, 9 Grosvenor Crescent, London SW1X 7EJ. Tel: 01–235 5454.

PHAB (Physically Handicapped and Able Bodied Clubs), 42 Devonshire Street, London W1N 1LN. Tel: 01–637 7475.
Organization providing social meetings, sport education, mainly

Appendices

1   Useful addresses and information

for the young disabled.

Queen Elizabeth's Foundation for the Disabled, Leatherhead,
   Surrey KT22 0BN. Tel: Oxshot 2204.
   General welfare, education, rehabilitation, recreation holidays.

The Royal Association for Disability and Rehabilitation (RADAR),
   25 Mortimer Street, London W1N 8AB. Tel: 01–637 5400.
   General information and advice on education employment, fund
   raising, etc.

Scottish Information Service for the Disabled, 18 Claremont
   Crescent, Edinburgh, Scotland EH7 4QD. Tel: 031–556 3882.
   General information.

Holidays and travel
Across Trust, c/o Trade and Technical Press Ltd, Crown House, Morden,
   Surrey.
   Have coach, ambulances to take disabled people on holiday.

Airline Users Committee, Space House, 43–59 Kingsway, London
   WC2B 6TE.
   Further information about air travel.

British Airports Authority, Press and Public Relations, Queen's
   Building, Heathrow Airport, London.
   Provide a free booklet giving details about facilities for disabled
   people at Heathrow (also available from the Disabled Living
   Foundation).

Cunard Steamship Company Ltd, Passenger Reservations, 15
   Regent Street, London SW1 4LY. Tel: 01–930 7890.
   Information on cruising.

Disabled Campers Club, 28 Coote Road, Bexleyheath, Kent DA7 4PR. Tel:
   01–303 0753.

Disabled Drivers' Association, Ashwellthorpe, Norwich NR16 1EX. Tel:
   Fundenhall 449.
   Own Ashwellthorpe Holiday Hotel. Produce the magazine *The Magic
   Carpet* free to members (4 issues a year).

Disabled Drivers' Motor Club, 39 Templewood, Ealing, London W13 8DU.
   Special concessions with car ferry crossings to the Continent, Isle of
   Wight and Channel Islands.

Appendices

1   Useful addresses and information

P and O Lines, P and O Building, Leadenhall Street, London EC3.
  Information on cruising.

The Royal Association for Disability and Rehabilitation (RADAR), 25
  Mortimer Street, London W1N 8AB. Tel: 01–637 5400.
  Provides a guide book called *Holidays for the Disabled* which lists all
  suitable accommodation. They also produce *Access to Public
  Conveniences*.

Scottish Tourist Board, 23 Ravelston Terrace, Edinburgh EH4 3EU.
  Publish information sheet for the disabled.

Wales Tourist Board, Welcome House, High Street, Llandaff, Cardiff CF5
  2YZ.
  Publish disabled visitor's guide to Wales.

Other organizations
British Orthopaedic Association, Royal College of Surgeons of England,
  35–43 Lincoln's Inn Fields, London WC2A 3PN. Tel: 01–405 3474.
  Professional society of orthopaedic surgeons.

British Society for Rheumatology, 3 St. Andrew's Place, Regent's Park,
  London NW1 4LE. Tel: 01–224 3739.
  Professional society of rheumatologists.

National Fund for Research into Crippling Diseases, Vincent House, 1
  Springfield Road, Horsham, W. Sussex RH12 2PN. Tel: Horsham
  64101.

The British Association of Occupational Therapists, 20 Rede Place, off
  Chepstow Place, London W2 4TU. Tel: 01–229 9738/9.
  Professional society of occupational therapists.

The Chartered Society of Physiotherapists, 14 Bedford Row, London
  WC1R 4ED. Tel: 01–242 1941.
  Professional society of physiotherapists.

REMAP, c/o British Council for Rehabilitation of the Disabled, Thames
  House North, Millbank, London SW1P 4QG.
  Panels of engineers — advise on adaptations and design new devices.

The Society for Back Pain Research, Department of Medical Biophysics,
  University of Manchester, Manchester M13 7PA.
  Organization of health professionals working in the field of back pain
  research.

Appendices

2 Further reading

Reference works

Dieppe P.A., Dogherty M., Macfarlane D. & Maddison P.J. (eds) (1985) *Rheumatological Medicine*. Churchill Livingstone, London.

Kelley W.N., Harris E.D., Ruddy S. & Sledge C.B. (eds) (1985) *Textbook of Rheumatology*. W.B. Saunders, Philadelphia.

McCarty D.J. (ed) (1985) *Arthritis and Allied Conditions*. Lea and Febiger, Philadelphia.

Scott J.T. (ed) (1986) *Copeman's Textbook on the Rheumatic Diseases*. 6th edn Churchill Livingstone, London.

Woolf A.D. & Dixon A.S. (1988) Practical Problems in Medicine: Osteoporosis a Clinical Guide. Martin Dunitz, London.

Journals

Arthritis and Rheumatism, 17 Executive Park Dr., Suite 480, Atlanta, Georgia 30329, USA.

Annals of the Rheumatic Diseases, British Medical Association, Tavistock Square, London WC1H 9JR, UK.

British Journal of Rheumatology, Baillière, Tindall, Vincent Square, London SW1 2PN, UK.

Journal of Rheumatology, 250 Bloor St E., Ste 401, Toronto M4W 3P2, Canada.

Rheumatic Disease Clinics of North America, W.B. Saunders, Philadelphia, USA.

Seminars in Arthritis and Rheumatism, Grune and Stratton Inc, PO Box 6280, Duluth, MN 55806, USA.

Index

Acquired immune deficiency syndrome (AIDS) 186
and arthritis 197
Acromioclavicular joint
arthritis 83, 84
injection 285
Acrosclerosis 143
Adhesive capsulitis 82, 84
Adson test 31–32, 92
Aids to daily living 259, 299–301
osteoarthritis 119
Aldolase, serum 50
Algodystrophy 82, 83, 84, 165, 184–185
Alkaline phosphatase, serum 50
Allis test 26
Allopurinol 156–157, 214, 252
Allowances for disabled 261
Amyloidosis 16, 91, 104, 124, 158, 202, 219–220, 267
Anaemia of chronic disease 52, 109–110
Analgesics 106, 111, 119, 162, 164, 181, 183, 209, 222
Ankle/foot
examination 28–29
joint injection 288–289
pain 11, 13–14
rheumatoid arthritis 99
surgery 266
Ankylosing spondylitis (AS) 4, 5, 7, 10, 16, 30, 42–43, 69, 77, 122–128
clinical features 72, 82, 123
investigations 62, 124–125
management 126–128, 241, 244
surgery 262, 263, 264
Antibiotics 141, 188, 189, 191, 192, 193
prophylactic 191
Anticardiolipin antibody (ACL) 46, 48, 141, 165
Anticoagulants 245, 265, 266
Antimalarials 14, 245–246
Antinuclear antibodies (ANA) 45–47, 101, 139, 141, 144, 146, 147, 148, 149, 203, 212
Antinuclear factor *see* Antinuclear antibodies
Arthrography 61, 83
Arthroscopy 83, 293–294
Aseptic necrosis 64, 138, 179–182

Azathioprine 106, 110, 130, 133, 140, 147, 156, 167, 209, 234, 252–253

Back pain 10–11, 69–76
Back strain, acute 30, 71, 75
Behçet's syndrome 4, 5, 7, 17, 18, 48, 220–221
Beighton scoring system 36
Bicipital tendinitis 23, 24, 82, 83
Biochemical tests 49–50, 51–58
Biopsies 266–267
Bisphosphonates 173,
Bone absorptiometry 63
Bone biopsy 294–296
Bone disease 50, 170–185
Bone fracture 198–199
Borellia burgdorferi 194
Bornholm disease 16
Brucellosis 8
Bunions 271
Bursal injection 289

C-reactive protein 42
Calcaneal bursitis 90
Calcaneal spurs 28, 271
Calcific tendinitis 82, 162–163
Calcinosis 22, 142
Calcitonin 173, 183
Calcium hydroxyapatite arthropathy 162–164
Calcium pyrophosphate deposition 158–162, 178
Capillaroscopy 37
Car conversion 302–303
Cardiovascular involvement 16
ankylosing spondylitis 123
Lyme disease 193–194
Reiter's disease 132, 133
rheumatic fever 229
rheumatoid arthritis 100, 101
Carpal tunnel injection 289, 291
Carpal tunnel syndrome 14, 21, 91–92, 219
Cervical radiculopathy 32, 33, 78
Cervical rib 92
See also Thoracic outlet syndrome
Cervical spondylosis 8, 9, 12, 78–79, 80
Chlemonucleolysis 76
Chlorambucil 106, 221, 255
Chloramphenicol 134, 193
Cholestyramine 223

309

Index

Chondrocalcinosis 57, 158, 161, 177, 200, 293
Chronic sprain syndrome 72
Churg–Strauss syndrome 15, 210–211
Clinical history 3–18
Colchicine 145, 153, 156, 161, 221, 222, 233
Colestipol 223
Complement deficiency 48–49
Complement measurement 48–49, 54
Computerized axial tomography *see* CT scan
Connective tissue disease 137–149, 252
Cord compression 10, 18
  cervical 78, 80, 100
Corticosteroids 14, 17, 107, 134, 136, 140, 141, 142, 147, 149, 153, 185, 186, 209, 218, 221, 232, 234, 250–251
  local injection 83, 84, 87–88, 89, 90, 91, 92, 93, 106, 109, 119, 120, 121, 126, 130, 133, 135, 161, 163, 167, 251, 279–292, 294
Cozen's test 22
Creatinine phosphokinase 50, 146
CREST syndrome 16, 142, 143
Cryoglobulin 49
Crystal arthropathy 51, 115, 121, 150–164
CT scan 62, 179
Cyclophosphamide 106, 140, 209, 212, 213, 215, 221, 254–255

Dapsone 232
de Quervain's tenosynovitis 21, 88
Dermatomyositis (DM) 15, 37, 43, 50, 146–147, 250
Diabetes 15, 73, 113, 115, 179, 187, 230, 268, 279
Dietary modification 272–275
Diffuse idiopathic skeletal hyperostosis (DISH) 73
Disc prolapse 10, 11, 14, 30, 71–72, 76, 78, 115, 264
  tests 32–33
'Dong diet' 273

Elbow
  examination 22
  injection 284–285
  nodule biopsy 266–267
  pain 8
  in rheumatoid arthritis 99
  surgery 263
Enthesitis 123
Enthesitis injection 291–292
Entrapment neuropathies 91–93
Eosinophilic fasciitis 145
Epiphyseal dysplasias 115
Erythrocyte sedimentation rate (ESR) 41–42
'Eskimo diet' 273
Essential cryoglobulinaemia 49
Examination, clinical 19–37
External ear involvement 16, 152
Eye involvement 7, 14, 16
  ankylosing spondylitis 123
  Behçet's syndrome 220
  juvenile ankylosing spondylitis 204
  juvenile chronic arthritis 201
  psoriatic arthropathy 129
  Reiter's syndrome 132, 133
  rheumatoid arthritis 99
  systemic lupus erythematosus 138
  Wegener's granulomatosis 211
  Whipple's disease 135

Facet joint arthritis 10, 78
Familial Mediterranean Fever 221–222
Felty's syndrome 45, 100, 111–112
Fibrositis 15, 85–87
Finkelstein's test 21, 88
Flexor tenosynovitis 87
  systemic lupus erythematosus 138, 139
Fluoride 173
Food intolerance 274–275
Fungal infections of joints 196–197

Gastrointestinal involvement 5–6, 16–17
  Behçet's syndrome 220
  Reiter's syndrome 131
  scleroderma 143, 144
  systemic lupus erythematosus 138
Generalized nodal osteoarthritis 113, 114
Giant cell arteritis (GCA) 12, 14, 17, 165–169

Index

Glenohumeral arthritis 82–83, 84
Gold 17, 106, 107, 108, 112, 130, 213, 214, 246–248
Gonococcal arthritis 5, 18, 58, 191–192
Gout 22, 28, 49, 103–104, 150–157
  acute 150, 153
  asymptomatic hyperuricaemia 150, 156
  chronic tophaceous 150, 152, 153
  diet and 154, 272–273
  intercritical 150
  long-term drug treatment 154–157
  renal involvement 152
  uricostatic drugs 154, 155
Guanethidine blockade 185

Haemarthrosis 199–200
Haematological tests 52–53
Haemochromatosis 4, 115–116
Haemophilia 199, 200
Hallux rigidus 271
Hand/wrist
  clinical examination 19–21
  injection 283–284
  osteoarthritis management 120
  pain 8, 9
  rheumatoid arthritis 98, 101
Henoch–Schönlein purpura 17, 18, 214
Hip
  dysplasia 4
  examination 24–26
  injection technique 285, 287
  osteoarthritis 114, 121
  pain 11, 12
  rheumatoid arthritis 99
  surgery 121, 127, 264–265
History taking 3–8
Homocystinuria 223
Hormone replacement 172
Hydralazine 7, 141
Hydrotherapy 257
Hydroxychloroquine 106, 107, 140, 147, 245–246
Hyperbetalipoproteinaemia 222, 223
Hyperlipoproteinaemia 222–223
Hypermobility 33, 36, 223–224
  Beighton scoring system 36
Hyperparathyroidism 177–179, 294
Hypertriglyceridaemia 222, 223
Hypertrophic pulmonary
  osteoarthropathy 224–225
Hyperviscosity syndrome 45

Idiopathic destructive arthritis 163–164
Immune complex assays 49
Indomethacin 12, 126, 153, 240, 244
Infection 51, 58
  joint and 186–197
  low back pain and 75
  radioisotope scan and 62
Inflammatory bowel disease 6, 7, 17, 43, 134–135, 239
Insocks 268
Intermittent hydrarthrosis 225–226
Ischial bursitis 89
Isoniazid 141

Jaccoud's arthritis 138, 229
Juvenile ankylosing spondylitis 204
Juvenile chronic arthritis 42, 201–204, 219
Juvenile monarthritis 205–206
Juvenile psoriatic arthritis 205
Juvenile rheumatoid arthritis 204–205

Kashin-Beck disease 115
Kawasaki's disease 209–210
Knee
  arthroscopy 293–294
  examination 26–27
  haemarthrosis 199–200
  injection 287–288
  osteoarthritis 115, 121
  pain 11, 13
  rheumatoid arthritis 99
  surgery 265–266
Kyphosis, thoracic 30

Laboratory tests 41–50
Laminectomy 76
Lateral epicondylitis 8, 22, 88, 291, 292
Lateral popliteal nerve compression 93
Latex text 43
Leg length measurement 25
Lindner's sign 33
Löfgren's syndrome 232–233
Lordosis, lumbar 30
Lumbar nerve root compression 36

311

Index

Lumbar spondylosis 71, 72
Lyme disease 18, 193—195
Magnetic resonance imaging (MRI) 63—65, 182
March fracture 198
Medial epicondylitis 8, 22, 88, 291, 292
Medial nerve compression *see* Carpal tunnel syndrome
Medical social worker 259—260
Meningococcal arthritis 192—193
Meralgia paraesthetica 25, 92—93
Metastatic deposits 10, 30, 74, 79, 198, 294
Methotrexate 106, 110, 130, 133, 147, 134, 253—254
Methylprednisolone 213, 251
Microscopic polyarteritis 48
Milgram test 33
Mixed connective tissue disease 46, 149
Mixed essential cryoglobulinaemia 215—216
Mononeuritis multiplex 15, 100, 207, 210, 211, 212
Morton's metatarsalgia 28, 93
Multicentric reticulohistiocytosis 226—227
Muscle biopsies 267

Neck
 acute strain 8, 9, 78, 80
 pain 8—10, 77—80
 rheumatoid arthritis 101, 102, 103
 surgery 262, 263—264
Nervous system involvement 12, 14—15
 ankylosing spondylitis 123—124
 Behçet's syndrome 220
 Lyme disease 193
 mixed essential cryoglobulinaemia 215
 rheumatoid arthritis 100
 Sjögren's syndrome 148
 systemic lupus erythematosus 138, 140
 Wegener's granulomatosis 211
 Whipple's disease 135
Neurological dermatomes 34, 35
Neuropathic joint disease 230—231
Neutrophil alkaline phosphatase antibody 48

Nifedipine 144
Non-steroidal anti-inflammatory drugs (NSAIDs) 7, 11, 12, 17, 72, 75, 80, 83, 239—245
 gastrointestinal bleeding 239, 244—245
 indications 106, 111, 119, 124, 126, 130, 133, 135, 139, 153, 154, 156, 161, 162, 182, 209, 218, 221, 222, 223, 225, 227, 229, 232, 233, 244
 toxicity 239, 240—241, 243—244

Occupational therapy 258—259
Olecranon bursitis 8, 89
Osgood—Schlatter syndrome 27
Osteoarthritis 4, 33, 57, 62, 103, 113—121, 181, 200, 223, 244, 293
 diet and 273
 local steroid injection 280, 284
 surgery 263
Osteogenesis imperfecta 223
Osteomalacia 62, 173—177, 198, 294
Osteonecrosis 82, 83, 179—182
Osteoporosis 10, 30, 62, 63, 74, 82, 99, 170—173, 177, 187, 198, 222, 294

Paget's disease 62, 63, 74, 182—184, 198, 294
Pelvic rock test 31
Penicillamine 17, 106, 107, 108, 145, 213, 247, 248—249
Penicillin 192, 213, 229
Phalen's test 21, 91
Phenylbutazone 18, 126, 242
Physiotherapy 83, 84, 108, 109, 119, 127, 133, 185, 189, 256—258
Pigmented villonodular synovitis 199, 227—228
Plant thorn synovitis 228
Plantar fasciitis 28, 123, 291
Plasma proteins 50
Plasma viscosity 42
Polyarteritis nodosa (PAN) 15, 207—209
Polymyalgia rheumatica 4, 7, 41, 165—167, 250
Polymyositis 50, 146—147
Prednisolone 84, 106, 140, 141, 147, 166—167, 168, 209, 211, 212, 215, 217, 250—251
Pre-patella bursitis 89

Index

Probenecid 155, 157
Probucol 223
Prosthetic joint infection 190–191
Pseudogout 116, 177
  acute 57, 158, 159–160, 161
Psoriatic arthropathy 103, 128–131, 253, 280
Purine-rich foods 154
Pyogenic arthritis, acute 186–189, 190
Pyrophosphate arthropathy 158, 159, 160–161, 280

Radiography 61, 262
Radioisotope bone scan 62, 83, 182
Reactive arthritis 131, 280
Rectal biopsy 267
Referred pain 75, 81, 86
Rehabilitation 256–261
Reiter's syndrome 4, 5, 6, 7, 17, 18, 28, 43, 131–133, 244, 253
Relapsing polychondritis 15, 16, 231–232
Renal involvement
  gout 152
  Henoch–Schönlein purpura 214
  hyperparathyroidism 177
  mixed essential cryoglobulinaemia 215, 216
  osteomalacia and 174
  scleroderma 143, 144–145
  Sjögren's syndrome 147–148
  systemic lupus erythematosus 138
  Wegener's granulomatosis 211
Repetitive strain injury 90
Respiratory involvement 16
  acrosclerosis 143
  ankylosing spondylitis 123
  rheumatoid arthritis 100, 101, 112
  Sjögren's syndrome 148
  systemic lupus erythematosus 138, 140, 141
  Wegener's granulomatosis 211
Reversed Lasegue test 33
Rheumatic fever 16, 17, 22, 41, 228–229
Rheumatoid arthritis (RA) 97–112
  anaemia and 109–110
  arthroscopy 293, 294
  clinical features 5, 8, 15, 16, 21, 22, 23, 28, 29, 82, 89, 90, 91, 98–100, 110–111, 112, 147, 199, 212–213, 219, 268, 280
  complications 104–105
  diet and 273–274
  drug treatment 106–108, 173, 239–254
  investigations 41, 42, 43, 45, 49, 57, 58, 100–102
  surgery 262, 263, 265
Rheumatoid factor (RF) 43–44, 97, 100, 101, 109, 116, 205, 212, 213, 215
Rheumatoid nodules 22, 99, 102
Rose–Waaler reaction 44
Rotator cuff 23, 24, 82, 83

Sarcoid arthropathy 232–234
Scaphoid fracture 198, 280
Schirmer's test 37, 148
Schober's test 32, 123
Scoliosis 30
Septic arthritis 8, 58, 62, 82, 104–105, 134, 191–195
Seronegative spondylarthropathies 8, 16, 122–136
Shoes 268, 269–271
Shoulder
  examination 22–24, 32
  injection 285, 287
  pain 81–84
  rheumatoid arthritis 99
  surgery 263
Shoulder–hand syndrome *see* Algodystrophy
Sjögren's syndrome 5, 7, 16, 17, 37, 47, 100, 147–149
Skin biopsy 267
Skin involvement 5, 17–18
  adult Still's disease 218
  Churg–Strauss syndrome 210
  gonococcal arthritis 192
  Kawasaki's disease 209
  Lyme disease 193
  polyarteritis nodosa 208, 209
  psoriatic arthropathy 128, 129
  Reiter's syndrome 132
  small vessel vasculitis 213, 214, 215
  systemic lupus erythematosus 137–138, 140
  Wegener's granulomatosis 211
Small vessel vasculitis 213, 214, 215
Social service resources 260

313

Index

Spinal stenosis 10, 11, 33, 62, 73, 76, 264
Spinal surgery 264
Spine examination 30–33
Spondylolisthesis 30, 72–73, 76, 264
Stevens–Johnson syndrome 18, 244
Still's disease
  adult 218
  juvenile *see* Juvenile chronic arthritis
Straight leg raising tests 32
Stress fracture 28, 198
Subacromial bursa injection 285
Sulindac 239, 240, 244
Sulphasalazine 106, 107, 110, 134, 249–250
Surgery 262–267
Sweet's syndrome 234–235
Synovial biopsy 267
Synovial fluid tests 51, 57–58, 61, 83, 160, 164
Systemic lupus erythematosus (SLE) 4, 5, 7, 16, 17, 18, 104, 137–142
  clinical features 15, 137–138, 139, 140, 147, 212–213
  drug treatment 139–140, 245, 250, 252, 254
  investigations 41, 43, 45, 46, 48, 49, 50, 139
  neonatal 142
  skin biopsy 267
Systemic sclerosis (SS) 5, 6, 7, 16, 17, 37, 43, 46, 142–145, 147, 268

Takayasu's arteritis 216–217
Tarsal tunnel syndrome 28, 93
Temporal artery biopsy 267

Temporomandibular joint injection 285
Tendon sheath injection 289
Tetracycline 136, 144, 195
  labelling 172, 175, 294
Thermography 62–63
Thomas' test 26
Thoracic outlet syndrome 31–32, 92
Tinel's test 21, 91
Torticollis 8, 78
Trendelenburg sign 25–26, 264
Triamcinolone 76, 126, 161, 251, 280, 281
Tuberculosis (TB) 5, 7, 30, 75, 58, 193–194, 293

Ulcerative colitis (UC) 134
Ulnar nerve entrapment 92
Uric acid, serum 49–50

Vasculitis 15, 17, 43, 49, 100, 106, 149, 207–212
  drug treatment 209, 211, 212, 213, 214, 215, 217, 250, 254
  necrotizing 207–212
Viral arthritis 5, 196–197

Wegener's granulomatosis 15, 48, 211–212
Whipple's disease 6, 17, 135–136
Wry neck 78, 80

Xanthomatosis 22
Xerostoma, drug-induced 148

Yergason's test 24, 82
Yersinia reactive arthritis 133–134